CONTENTS

Preface

1. **Diagnosis of Diagnostic Methods**
2. **Laboratory Tests in Oral Diagnosis and Oral Medicine**
3. **Developmental Disorder**
4. **Infections**
5. **Dental Caries**
6. **Diseases of Pulp and Periapical Tissues**
7. **Injuries of Oral Cavity: Repair and Alteration of the Teeth**
8. **Mucocutaneous Disorders**
9. **Vesiculobullous Disorders**
10. Facial Pain and Nerve Disorders
11. **Cysts of Oral Cavity**
12. **Pre-malignant Conditions and Lesions**
13. **Tumors**
14. Syndromes of Head and Neck
15. References

Preface

Short question answers are as important as essay questions. These question answers are used to assess knowledge in VIVA examinations and competitive examinations. This book is an attempt to compile questions which require short answers. However readers are advised to read standard textbooks for detailed answers and references.

Syndromes form an important part in any of the textbook. Keeping this in view for important and significant syndromes exhibiting the oral manifestations have been included for easy and ready reference.

It is hoped that the readers will find this book useful. They are free to write their opinion and comments to the author, which may help in bringing out an improved second edition.

I wish to express my gratitude and sincere pranama to His Holiness Jagadguru Sri Sri Shivarathree Deshikendra Mahaswamiji for providing me the opportunity to serve this institution and continue to gain the experience and knowledge.

Many of my colleaques have helped me in preparation of script, proof reading and corrections. I wish to record my sincere thanks to Dr. Karthikeya Patil, Dr. (Mrs) Mahima Patil, Dr. Raghavendra Kini, Dr. B.N. Praveen, Dr. Rupam Sinha, Dr. Veena and Dr. Sujatha for their help.

I also place on record the help and co-operation extended by Mr. Gururaj and Mr. Arun of CAM Zone, Mysore.

Dr. N. S. Yadav

1.

DIAGNOSIS AND DIAGNOSTIC METHODS

Q1. What is diagnosis ?
Ans. Diagnosis is identification of disease or abnormality by use of scientific knowledge and methods and correlation of information thus obtained.

Q2. Name different types of diagnosis ?
Ans. Provisional diagnosis, Tentative diagnosis, Clinical diagnosis, Spot diagnosis, Differential diagnosis, Radiological diagnosis, Histopathological diagnosis, Laboratory diagnosis and Therapeutic diagnosis.

Q3. What is the provisional diagnosis ?
Ans. Provisional diagnosis or clinical diagnosis or tentative diagnosis, are the diagnosis arrived at from the findings of history and clinical examination. It is only clinical impression and may require additional tests for confirmation.

Q4. What is therapeutic diagnosis ?
Ans. Therapeutic diagnosis is diagnosis arrived after the beneficial effect of the therapy is known. In certain cases like trigeminal neuralgia, the clinical findings may not be typical of disease hence administration of treatment (carbamezapine) may be done. If the drug is found effective the diagnosis may be confirmed.

Q5. What is the importance of diagnosis ?
Ans. Diagnosis is important as it identifies, and indicates, nature of etiological factors, nature of pathological process

involved or the tissues involved in the condition. This information is essential for treatment planning and prognosis.

Q6. What is differential diagnosis ?
Ans. Differential diagnosis is a term used to differentiate the multiple conditions from one to another which may present few common and similar signs and symptoms.

Q7. What is the importance of differential diagnosis ?
Ans. Differential diagnosis enables one to arrive at correct diagnosis after eliminating other conditions. This will help us in planning the treatment correctly. Gingival enlargements may be caused by various etiological factors including vitamin 'C' deficiency, by local irritants, as side effect to use of antihypertensive drug or due to leukemia. These need different treatment approach. The correct diagnosis arrived after eliminating other causes in differential diagnosis, the management becomes easy.

Q8. What is prognosis ?
Ans. The prognosis is the term used to describe the progress and outcome of the disease.

Q.9. What are the basic requirements one is required to possess to be good diagnostician ?
Ans. The good diagnostician should have basic knowledge of normal anatomy, histology and physiology of the parts of the body and pathological chares occurring due to various diseases in these tissues and should be able to correlate the findings in proper prospective.

Q10. What is comprehensive diagnosis ?
Ans. The comprehensive diagnosis is term, sometimes used for identifying the diseases or abnormalities which may or may not cause acute symptoms. This includes the diagnosis of all the problems after detailed examinations of all the tissues.

Q11. What is emergency diagnosis ?
Ans. In case of accidental injuries, due to automobile or otherwise, the priority is given for emergency management on the clinical impression obtained from short examination without waiting for detailed examination and investigation. Diagnosis made in such situation is referred as emergency diagnosis.

Q12. Which is the first step in diagnosis ?
Ans. The diagnostic process ideally should commence with arrival of patient with close observation as to the general behaviour, gait and facial expression. These observations may help in assessing the psychological buildup and suffering and also facies peculiar to certain diseases may be observed in such patients.

Q13. Name the steps in recording of history of patient during clinical examination.
Ans. (1) Recording of personal data (2) Chief complaint (3) History of present illness. (4) History of past dental illness (5) Past medical history (6) Family history (7) Social (8) Occupational and (9) Personal history.

Q14. Which are the particulars required in personal biodata ?
Ans. (1) Name (2) Age (3) Sex) (4) Address (5) Personal identification marks (6) Occupation.
The above particulars are essential to establish identity of individual, communication and diagnosis of certain disorders.

Q15. What is the importance of recording of name of individual in biodata?
Ans. Name contributes to individual's personality and identification. It is essential for identification, communication and medico-legal problems. Further more if the doctor addresses the patient with his/her name, while recording history and initial examination, it helps in development of good rapport between doctor and patient.

Q16. How does the age of the patient helps in oral diagnosis ?

Ans. Age of patient is an important aspects of biodata. It may help in diagnosis of certain disorders which are more common in particular age groups. Primary viral infections occur in children. Unerupted permanent maxillary tooth may be normal physiological finding in the age group of 5 to 6 years however same finding shall be considered pathological if it is seen after the age of 8 years.

Q17. How does the occupation of an individual helps in diagnosis ?

Ans. Few diseases/ abnormalities are common and typical to certain occupations. Notch like attrition of incisal edges of anterior teeth is seen in tailors who hold the needles in that particular area. Erosions of teeth are common in individuals working in factories with predominant acid fumes. Presence of metallic line (lead line) in gingival is more likely to appear in workers in lead factories and workers in printing presses.

Q18. Give the importance of history of present illness in diagnosis.

Ans. History of present illness shall include in sequence the particulars of events like mode of onset, signs and symptoms during its progress to present stage. Thus behaviour pattern may indicate the nature of disease and help in diagnosis. Occurrence of swelling after pain at the site usually indicate the inflammatory disease.

Q19. Give the importance of medical history.

Ans. In medical history much importance have to be given to serious chronic diseases more particularly like, tuberculosis, diabetes, hypertension, rheumatic fever and bleeding disorders etc. These diseases may not only alter or influence the cause of oral and dental diseases but also may influence the treatment procedures. Special extra care may be required in such situations.

Q20. How does the "negative findings" help in diagnosis?
Ans. Many a times recording of negative findings in answers are important in diagnosis. Absence of watery discharge at the time of meals, from the sinus at the angle of mandible at once rules out the presence of parotid fistula.

Q21. What are the components of patient's history and examination ?
Ans. The components of patient's history include collection, compilation and analysis of information pertaining to routine personal data, chief complaint, history of present illness, history of past dental and medical illness and their treatments, history of any hospitalization history of any untoward reactions to drugs including allergies, family history, social and occupational particulars, review of systems, and physical examination of orofacial tissue in general and tissues related to the complaint in particular.

Q22. What are the steps in the examination ?
Ans. Examination shall include examination and local examination. The examination method include inspection, palpation, and auscultation.

Q23. Give the components of examination procedure.
Ans. The examination procedure shall include (1) examination and recording of Vital signs like pulse, temperature, respiratory rate and blood pressure (2) Examination of regional lymyh nodes of orofacial region (3) Examination of head, neck and oral cavity and (4) examination of nervous, muscular and salivary glandular function.

Q24. What is the basic principle in examination of orofacial tissue ?
Ans. Examination should be done in systematic order, commencing the examination of parts of one side and proceeding to other. This shall include extra oral and intra oral examination. Examination in systematic order eliminates the chances of missing of examination of particular region.

Q25. What is lesion ?
Ans. Tissue alterations produced by disease process or abnormalities are referred to as lesions.

Q26. What is dysfunctions ?
Ans. Dysfunctions is defect or alteration in functioning of organ or tissue.

Q27. What are the significance of clinical manifestations.
Ans. The diseases or abnormalities may cause alterations or changes in structure of tissues (lesions) or may cause alterations in functioning of tissue or organ. These alterations manifest as changes in clinical appearance and behaviour.

Q28. What is the significance of systemic disease in orofacial disorders ?
Ans. The systemic diseases effecting heart, cardiovascular system, lymphatic system, blood, gastrointestinal system and excretory system may influence occurrence, progress and management of orofacial disorders.

Q29. What are the conditions, which are diagnosed mostly from findings of history rather than clinical findings ?
Ans. Neuralgias are diagnosed based mostly on findings of history rather than clinical examination findings. Clinical examination of parts is usually done to eliminate possible other causes.

Q30. What is SOAP evaluation ?
Ans. SOAP evaluation, is the evaluation and management of condition based on findings. 'S' stands for recording of subjective symptoms as given by patient. 'O' stands for objective signs obtained b the examiner. 'A' stands for analysis of the above data and 'P' stands for planning of management.

Q31. Mention few symptoms which may be indicative of cardiovascular disease.

Ans. Chest pain on exertion indicates angina pectoris. Edematous swellings of extremities and breathing discomfort also may indicate congestive heart failure.

Q32. Mention few symptoms which may be indicative of pulmonary disease.

Ans. Breathlessness, painful breathing, continuous and chronic cough, productive cough associated with pus or blood are the few symptoms which may be indicative of pulmonary diseases. These patients require further evaluation.

Q33. Mention the symptoms of some gastrointestinal diseases.

Ans. Pain in abdomen, persistent vomiting, frequent productive belching, blood in stools, diarrhea, are the few symptoms of G.I. tract diseases.

Q34. What are the symptoms of liver disease ?

Ans. Fullness of abdomen, loss of appetite, bleeding tendency and epigastric pain one hour after eating fatty foods etc.

Q35. What are the different immunological disorders ?

Ans. Immunological disorders could be either due to immune deficiency, hypersensitivity, or autoimmunity.

Q36. Which form of gingivitis is associated with chewing gum ?

Ans. Systemic or local use of different therapeutic drugs, variety of materials, jewellery, commercial skin products and denture material etc.

Q37. Which form of gingivitis is associated with chewing gum?

Ans. Plasma cell gingivitis is found in individuals who use chewing gum regularly.

Q38. What are the symptoms which may be indicative of endocrinal disorders ?

Ans. Unusual pattern of growth, uusual pattern of eruption of teeth, intolerance to mild temperature changes, excessive urination, excessive thirst, excessive appetite, pigmentation of skin and changes in secondary sexual characteristics, are the few symptoms which may require detail investigation of endocrinal disorders.

Q39. Mention few symptoms associated with blood disorders.

Ans. Constant fatigue may indicate anemia. Recurrent infections and unproductive cough may be the result of disorders of white blood cells. Echymosis, petechical hemorrhagic spots may indicate thrombocytopenia.

Q40. What is schirmer's test ?

Ans. Schirmer test is the test for measuring the lacrimation.

Q41. Describe schirmer's test.

Ans. Test is performed by hooking a 3 mm. wide strip of filter paper in the lower conjunctival fornix and measuring the length of moisten of strip. In individuals with normal lacrimation, about 15 mm of strip becomes moist in one minute.

Q42. What is paraesthesia ?

Ans. Paraesthesia is a term used to indicate altered sensation.

Q43. What is Formication ?

Ans. Formication is the term used to describe the sensory feeling which is described as experience of worms creeping below the skin. This is a form of paraesthesia.

Q44. What does anesthesia of part indicate ?

Ans. Anaesthesia of the area indicates loss of sensation either due to compression of sensory nerve or discontinuity of sensory nerve.

Q45. What is neuramatesis ?
Ans. Cutting of nerve which causes discontinuity is referred to as neuramatesis.

Q46. What is neuropraxia ?
Ans. Neuropraxia is the term used the describe the compression of nverve or partial cutting of the nerve.

Q47. What are the symptoms associated with central nervous system abnormalities ?
Ans. Persistent and chronic headache, syncope, vertigo, ataxia and diplopia.

Q48. Mention the methods of examination.
Ans. They are visual (inspection), palpation and functional evaluation of the part and transillumination.

Q49. How does the transillumination helps in examination of orofacial region ?
Ans. Transillumination test relies on the passage of light through relatively thin and translucent tissues thus helping in diagnosing the contents of swelling. Transillumination test can also be used to study maxillary sinusitis. Patient is placed in dardened room and an intense light cource is placed intraorally with patient's lip closed. The tissues overlying the normal maxillary sinus exhibits a dull glow, while congestion, presence of pus of fluid or abnormal soft tissue within the sinus blocks the diffusion of light.

Q50. What is fluctuation test ?
Ans. Fluctuation test is done to find the contents of large swelling.

Q51. Describe the method of fluctuation test.
Ans. Fluctuation test is done by placing finger of one hand on one aspect of swelling and finger of another hand on opposite aspect at a distant place. Then slow pressure in applied on one side. The pressure causes displacement of fluid and the movement of fluid is transmitted to other end and perceived by the finger on opposite side. Then it is

called positive fluctuation test. This indicatres presence of fluid. This is negative if the content of swelling is made up of soft tissue.

Q52. What is paget's test ?
Ans. Pagets test is done to find out the contents in smaller swellings.

Q53. Describe paget's test.
Ans. Page's test is done by exerting pressure with one finger over the smaller swelling. If the serlling contains fluid, the pressure of finger causes the fluid to displace to periphery thus increasing the pressure at the periphery. This changes consistency at the periphery. Thus change, at the periphery when pressure is applied at centre is referred as positive pagets test.

Q54. What is the diference between bimanual and bidigital palpation ?
Ans. **Bimanual palpation is performed with the hands while bidigital palpation is performed with two fingers.**

Q55. Write the procedure of bimanual palpation.
Ans. Bimanual palpation is performed with both the hands. One hand is used to manipulate and palpate the tissues while the other hand is used to support the structures from opposite side. This helps in trapping the tissues in between both the hand for better appreciation. This method is utilized for palpation of soft tissues of floor of the mouth.

Q56. Write the procedure for bidigital palpation.
Ans. This is similar to bimanual palpation. However fingers are used. One finger is used to manipulate and palpate the tissues while other finger is used to support. Bidigital palpation is usually done for thin tissues like lips and cheeks.

Q57. What is bony hardness?
Ans. Bony hard is a feeling to pressure. It is rigid, unyielding and hard feeling similar to bone indicating calcification or mineralization.

Q58. What is induration?
Ans. Induration is feeling of hardness but has very little y yielding. There is no rigidit as associated with bone. It is usually associated with malignant neoplasmas and indicates infiltration into deeper structures. It is similar to hard, solid rubber ball.

Q59. What is firm consistency?
Ans. Tissues having firm consistency yield to pressure little more than indicated masses. However there is minimal alteration in shape of growth, tissue or organ.

Q60. What is balanching?
Ans. Blanching is a term used to describe the changes of colored tissues or lesion which turn pale on pressure. Lesions and tumors of wascular in origin, will become pale when compressed due to escape of blood into deeper tissues and the lesions regain the original red or blue colour when pressure is released and blood flows back to the lesion.

Q61. What is pitting?
Ans. Pitting is the term used to describe the condition when tissue yield slightly to pressure but regain the shape after release of pressure.

Q62. What is tenderness?
Ans. Tenderness invariably indicates inflammatory conditions.

Q63. What does tenderness indicate?
Ans. Tenderness invariably indicates inflammatory conditions.

Q64. Mention a painful condition which is relieved on pressure unlike tenderness.
Ans. Headache. Relief from headache occurs with pressure.

Q65. What is diascopy ?
Ans. Blanching elicited by use of glass slide to apply pressure on small vascular lesions. Pressure is applied with glass slide and change of color is observed through glass slide.

Q66. Mention the procedure to test the taste sensation.
Ans. Taste sensations are tested by using solutions containing different agents preferably without smell. Four distinctive tasting substances are used. Sweet solution, salt solution, acid solution such as vinegar, and peppermint solutions are used. The patient, is asked to protrude tongue. The surface is touched with cotton pellet soaked in different solutions. The patients response is noted.

Q67. What is probing ?
Ans. Probing is the procedure to elicit information about surface continuity or tract continuity and extent of damage.

Q68. What are the types of probing ?
Ans. Soft tissue probing and Hard tissue probing.

Q69. Write the indication of soft tissue probing ?
Ans. Soft tissue probing is done by thin blunt canula like probes to study the location and extent of sinus tracts or fistula tracts. These are also indicated in study of patency, blocking of salivary gland ducts. Blunt periodontal probes are used to probe and measure thedepth of periodontal pockets.

Q70. Mention the indication of probing of hard tissues.
Ans. Probing on hard tissues is usually carried out to examine the teeth. Half round probes, and right angle probes with sharp edges are used to probe and diagnose the surface defects, crevices, pit and fissures on the teeth.

Q71. What is the test for functions of salivary glands ?
Ans. Function of salivary gland is assessed by the quantity and is assessed by the quantity and quality of saliva.

Q72. Mention the test for salivary flow.

Ans. Slivary flow can be observed by observing the amount of flow from the ductal opening. The area of ductal opening is dried with cotton and then evidence of flow will be visible with appearance of drops of saliva discharging from ductal opening. Sometimes various items of food which stimulate the salivary secretion are used for stimulation. Saliva also can be collected with the help of canula and suction cup.

Q73. Mention the types of intraoral mirrors.

Ans. Intraoral mirror could be plane or concave.

Q74. Mention the uses of intraoral mirror ?

Ans. Intraoral mirrors are used to visualize the tissue or teeth indirectly. Concave mirrors give magnified view. These can also be used as retractors of tissues like tongue and cheek during examination. Opposite end of the mirror handle which is blunt and slender is used to percuss the teeth for eliciting tendencess.

Q75. What are the disclosing solutions ?

Ans. Disclosing solutions are the solutions containing iodine and when applied on tooth surface will stain the areas of location of dental plaque.

Q76. What is pulp testing ?

Ans. Pulp tests are either based on response to thermal or electrical stimulations.

Q77. What are different methods of pulp tests ?

Ans. Pulp tests are either based on response to thermal or electrical stimulations.

Q78. Describe methods of thermal pulp test ?
Ans. They are either cold or hot. Ice or cotton pellet sprayed with ethyl chloride is applied on the dried tooth surface and response is compared with same tooth on other side. Similarly for heat test, warmed gutta percha stick is applied to dried surface to elicit the response.

Q79. Describe the method of electrical pulp test.
Ans. Electrical pulp testing is done by battery operated devices called "pulp tester". Mild electrical impulses are passed by keeping the tip of pulp tester on the dried tooth surface. The tip of pulp tester is coated with conductor like tooth paste for better conduction. Response to the stimulation is evaluated to assess the condition of the pulp.

Q80. What are the contraindications of electrical pulp tester ?
Ans. Electrical pulp testing is contraindicated in patients using pacemaker.

Q81. What are the methods of examination and assessment of occlusion ?
Ans. Occlusion of teeth can be studied by clinical examination and by the use of articulating paper to study the cuspal contact areas. Occlusion can also be studied and analysed by preparing plaster cast and mounting them on articulator.

Q82. Which is the commonest and most effectively used diagnostic aid ?
Ans. The most common and most effective diagnostic tool is radiographic examination.

Q83. What are different radiographic methods useful in oral diagnosis ?
Ans. 1. Plane radiographic examination using both intra oral and extra oral techniques.
2. Radiographs using contrast media.
3. Specialised techniques.

Q84. Which is the radiographic technique in which x-ray source is used but not the x-ray films to record the image ?

Ans. It is radiovisiography in which the x-rays are used as source but the image is visualized on screen (monitor) and the images can be printed on paper.

Q85. What are advantages of radiovisiography over regular radiographs ?

Ans. Amount of radiation required to produce the images in radiovisiography is very much less. The images can be produced instantly and do not require long time as required for processing of films. Contrast and density can be adjusted on monitor. The required area can be enlarged to four times for better visualization.

Q86. What are the different techniques of intraoral radiography?

Ans. Intraoral radiographic techniques include periapical radiographs, bite-wing radiographs, occlusal radiographs and radiovisiography.

Q87. What are the different extraoral projections ?

Ans. The extraoral proections can be taken in posteroanterior, anteroposterior, submento vertex, lateral directions. These can be taken either for whole skull or for parts of skull (sinuses, jaws etc.). The other extraoral projections are orthopantomograph and tomography.

Q88. Mention few indications where contrast media or agents are used in orofacial radiology.

Ans. Contrast media containing iodine are used for sialography. Gutta percha cones are used as contrast agents to study intraoral sinuses and depth of periodontal pockets and alveolar bone loss. Reamers are used to measure the root canal. Needle or pins are used to localize broken and embedded instruments or burs in soft tissues.

Q89. What are the specialized imaging techniques ?
Ans. The various imaging techniques include tomography, computerized tomography, magnetic resonance imaging and sonography.

Q90. What is chachexia ?
Ans. Cachexia is severely decreased tissue and organ mass resulting from servere malnutrition or from servere debilitating disease.

Q91. What are the different body builds in different individuals ?
Ans. Depending on skeletal and muscular build, the individuals are classified into four groups. They are asthenic, sthenic, hypersthenic, and pyknic. Asthenic individuals are slender, and have less than average mass of skeletal and muscular. Sthenic person is well proportioned with average build of bone and muscles development. The Hypersthenic person exhibits heavy bone and muscular development.
The pyknic persons have excessive fat than bone and muscle tissue. They appear round, soft and heavy.

Q92. What is aphasia ?
Ans. Aphasia is inability to accomplish proper verbal expression. It could be total or partial.

Q93. What is hypertelorism?
Ans. Hypertelorism is the increased distance between two eyes. It is the feature of some developmental disorders.

Q94. What are the parameters in assessing the function of temporomandibular joint ?
Ans. There are five components or parameters in assessing the function of ttemporo mandibular joints. They are palpation of condyle during opening and closing, determination of maximum opening, observation of lateral opening and closing and examination of muscles of mastication for tenderness and other abnormality and finally observation of clicking sound either with or without the aid of stethoscope.

Q95. What is average opening of the jaw bones ?
Ans. Opening of jaw bones or mouth is measured by interincisal distance between upper and lower central incisors. Average intercical edge distance is male is 4.5 to 5 cm and in female it is 3.5 to 4 cm.

Q96. What is anosmia ?
Ans. Anosmia is loss of sense of smell.

Q97. What is Romberg test ?
Ans. Romberg test is the test to evaluate the functioning of vestibulocochlear nerve. This nerve helps in maintaining proper gait and balance. Romberg test is done by making the person stand with eyes closed and hands extended. If person is able to stand for sometime ti is positive for normal functioning of nerve.

Q98. What is clubbing of fingers ?
Ans. Clubbing of fingers is thickening of distal ends of fingers. Generalized clubbing of all fingers usually indicates cardiovascular or cardiopulmonary disorders.

Q99. What is Koilonychia ?
Ans. Koilonychia is term used to describe dry, dull colored and spoon shaped nails. It is most often seen in iron deficiency anemia.

Q100. Which normal variations of buccal mucosa are likely to be mistaken for diseases ?
Ans. Presence of ectopic sebaceous glands (Fordyce spots) and prominent white mucosal line corresponding to occlusal plane (Linea alba buccalis) and prominent and enlarged opening of stenson duct.

Q101. What is papule ?
Ans. Papule is small, pin head sized well circumscribed, elevated, solid lesion of mucosa or the skin. It measures less than 2 mm in diameter.

Q102. What is nodule ?
Ans. Nodule is well circumscribed, solid mass of skin or mucosa and measuring more than 2 mm in diameter.

Q103. What is auspitz sign ?
Ans. Auspitz sign is seen in skin lesions of psoriasis. The sliklesions present with htin mica like scales. If the scales are removed, tiny bleeding points are disclosed underneath. This is called auspitz sign.

Q104. What is plaque ?
Ans. Solid, raised, flat surfaced patches over skin or mucosa and measuring about 1 cm or more are called plaques.

Q105. What is macule ?
Ans. Macule is well circumscribed area of altered color over mucosa or skin and which is not raised above adjacent area on skin or mucosa.

Q106. What is vesicle ?
Ans. Vesicle is elevated, circumscribed lesion of skin or mucosa containing fluid. It is less than 1 cm isn diameter.

Q107. What is bulla ?
Ans. Bulla is blister like lesion which is elevated, and well demarcated lesions containing fluid and measuring more than 1 cm in diameter.

Q108. What is an erosion ?
Ans. Erosion is moist, red lesion of skin or mucosa caused by loss of superficial cell layers of epithelium.

Q109. What is an ulcer ?
Ans. An ulcer is lesion caused by break in continuity of epithelium due to molecular disintegration of cells.

Q110. What are petechiae ?
Ans. Petechiae are the flat reddish to purple lesions caused by blood leaking out from blood vessels below the skin. They are less than 2 mm in diameter.

Q111. What is ecchymosis ?
Ans. Ecchymosis is a larger area of blood leaking from the blood vessels below epithelium. These eiscoloured areas measure more than 2 mm to even few centimeters.

Q112. What are the methods or parameters which are considered in deciding the association of microorganisms with disease?
Ans. Microbial association with the disease may be assessed by any of the following (i) characteristic features of the disease (ii) isolation of organisms from the lesions (iii) microbial pure culturing from the swabs or contents of lesions (iv) recognizing the microorganisms from biopsy tissues and (v) estimating the concentration of specific antibodies either in blood, serum, or saliva.

Q113. What is serology ?
Ans. Serology refers to the measurement of antibodies and other substances that increase in concentration of serum (saliva and other body fluids are also include), following exposure to infective agent or noninfective antigenic agent.

Q114. Write general characteristics of viral infection ?
Ans. Virus infection may be suspected if any of the following signs and symptoms are found. Popular rash, vesicular eruptions, crop of multiple ulcers, relative lymphocytosis without significant leukocytosis, atypical lymphocytes, fever, malaise and muscular pains, gastrointestinal disturbances and lymphadenitis atypical of local disorders.

Q115. What is Schick test ?
Ans.   Schick test is the skin test which is performed to find out susceptibility of a person to Diphteria.

Q116. Describe the procedure of schick test.
Ans.   0.2 ml of diphtheria toxin is injected intradermally on left forearm and 0.2 ml of inactivated toxin (inactivated at 700C for 30 minutes) is injected intradermally on right forearm. Readings or changes are recorded after one, four and seven days. The types of reactions may determine susceptibility. In positive reactions an area of erythema and swelling appears at the site of inoculation of toxin within 24 to 48 hours and reaching maximum size of 5 cm in about a week. There is no reaching at the site of injection of inactivated toxin. In negative cases there is no reaction on either sites.
In few case the erythema and swelling may appear which regresses within 3 to 4 days indicating false reaction.

Q117. What is Kveimil Sitzbach test ?
Ans.   Kveim siltzbach test is an intracutaneous test for diagnosis of Sarcoidosis. It is performed by intradermal injection of suspension of human known sarcoidal tissue. In positive cases, nodular growth appears at the site of inoculation. Biopsy findings of nodule may be similar to sarcoidosis.

Q118. What are the types of fissured tongues ?
Ans.   Fissured tongue or scrotal tongue is classified depending on directions of fissures. These are foliaceous, cerebriform and transverse. However in few cases the fissures do not follow any specific pattern.

Q119. What is "Cupid's bow" lip ?
Ans.   Developmental disorder of lip exhibiting double lip appearance. The lip is divided into two by horizontal fissure. However it is not prominenet when lip is in relaxed position. Involved upper lip is tensed, the double lip resembles "cupid's bow".

Q120. What is lock jaw ?

Ans. Lock jaw is term used to describe the trismus caused by Tetanus. Facies in tetanus is described as "Risus Sardonicus". This is due to rigidity of facial muscles.

Q121. Which disease is charactersied by typical facies "Hebra Nose"?

Ans. Chronic unusual infection, Rhinoscleroma in which granulomatous, and nodular lesions are found in upper respiratory tract. The proliferative masses in nose produce a typical facies which is described as "Herba Nose".

Q122. What do "cafe au lait" spots indicate ?

Ans. "Café au lait" spots are irregularly pigmented melanotic spots of light brown color. These are found in polyostotic fibrous dysplasia.

Q123. What is patch test ?

Ans. Patch test is performed to test hypersensitivity of different agents (Like denture material and food stuffs).

2.

LABORATORY TESTS IN ORAL DIAGNOSIS AND ORAL MEDICINE

Q1. What is biopsy ?
Ans. Biopsy is the procedure to obtain the tissue from the body for microscopic study.

Q2. Mention the different types of biopsy ?
Ans. Incisional biopsy, Excisional biopsy, Punch biopsy, Aspiration biopsy, Bone marrow biopsy and Exfoliative cytolofical biopsy.

Q3. What is the incisional biopsy ?
Ans. Incisional biopsy is the term used to describe biopsy procedure when only a part of pathological tissue is removed. This is indicated in large and deep lesions and also in lesions with doubtful diagnosis.

Q4. What is the excisional biopsy ?
Ans. Excisional biopsy is indicated in small lesions and also benign lesions which can be accessible to surgery easily. The procedure is to excise the lesion completely and send for histopathological study.

Q5. What is punch biopsy ?
Ans. Punch biopsy is a type of incisional biopsy wherein a part of abnormal tissue is obtained by means of instrument called punch. However, the specimen thus obtained is very small.

Q6. **what are the different methods of processing the tissue for microscopic study ?**
Ans. (1) Paraffin embedding, (2) parlodion embedding. (3) Frozen sections and (4) Ground sections sections.

Q7. **what is fixing the tissue specimen ?**
Ans. Tissue specimen which are obtained through biopsy are to be preserved before further processing. The preservation maintains the cellular organelles and structure in same state and does not allow autolysis. This procedure is referred to as "Fixation of tissue" or preservative.

Q8. **What is the normal fixative used ?**
Ans. 10% neutral formalin is the routine fixative.

Q9. **What is the duration of fixing a tissue ?**
Ans. It may vary from few hours to few weeks. It depends on size and density of tissue. Small size tissue and less dense tissue take less time for infiltration of preservative into the deeper parts of tissue.

Q10. **What are the precautions to be taken while obtaining biopsy specimen ?**
Ans. (1) Local anaesthic shall be injected around the lesion and not into the lesion.
(2) Local application which stain the tissue (Gen tian violet) shall not be used, as they may interfere with other stains.
(3) Sharp instrument shall be used to cut the tissue. Blunt instrunts will cause tissue destruction.
(4) Electosurgery shall not be used as the margins of specimen are destroyed.
(5) The specimen shall be preserved immediately in proper fixative in wide mouth jars or botties.

Q96. **What are the limitations of serological examinations ?**
Ans. The limitations or disadvantage of serological examinations are that they usually provide only retrospective diagnosis. The tests are negative in initial or acute stage as the

antibodies are not present. The antibodies develop later, hence, the tests become positive in later period of disease. Added to this the serological tests are very expensive.

Q97. What is ELISA test ?
Ans. It is a serological test for detection of viral diseases. It is Enzyme Linked Immuno Sorbent Assay test, in which either peroxide or alkaline phosphatase in used as the label and antigen is measured spectrophotometrically after incubation with a color producing substrate specific for the enzyme.

Q98. What is radioimmunoassay test ?
Ans. Radioimmunoassay is a test in which isotopes are used as a label and antigen is measured by gamma counter.

Q99. Which isotope is used in RIA test ?
Ans. I^{125} is used as a label in radioimmunoassay test.

Q100. Which tests are useful in diagnosis of infectious mononucleosis ?
Ans. PaulBunnell test, Davidson test which is a modification of Paul Bunnell test and rapid qualitative agglutination tests like Mono test are useful in diagnosis of infectious mononucleosis.

Q101. What are the warm agglutinins and cold agglutinins ?
Ans. The antibodies directed against red blood cells may exhibit maximal reactivity either at incubation temperature of 37^0C or at cold refrigerator temperature of 4^0C. The former antibodies are referred as warm agglutinins and latter are referred as cold agglutinins.

Q102. What is the normal T4 lymphocyte count ?
Ans. The normal T4 lymphocyte count ranges from 800 per cmm to 1200 cmm.

3.
DEVELOPMENTAL DISORDERS

Q1. What is the development disorder ?
Ans. The developmental disorder is the abnormality, defect or disturbance which occur during developmental stage of tissue or organ.

Q2. What is congenital disorder ?
Ans. The congenital disorder is the abnormality or defect which occurs during development process in intrauterine period. The manifestation may be visible at the time of birth or later period when the effected tissues become visible (Teeth).

Q3. What is inherited disorder?
Ans. The disorders or abnormalities which are transmitted through genes to off springs in next or subsequent generation.

Q4. What is genetic disorder ?
Ans. The disorder or abnormality which is caused by gene abnormality or mutation.

Q5. What is sex linked disease ?
Ans. The disorder or diseases which are caused by genetic aberrations of sex chromosomes.

Q6. What is difference between congenital and inherited disease ?
Ans. Congenital disease is caused by changes occurring during intrauterine life, and need neither be due to genetic abnormality nor carried forward in next generations.

Q7. What is the principle of dominance in inherited diseases ?

Ans. If the two members of a given pair of individuals with contrasting characters are brought together in a cross, there is a decided difference in the ability of these character to be expressed, in the resulting offspring. The one of the characters may appear in immediate offspeing whereas other characters which are not expressed, are ot completely eliminated and they may be manifested in subsequent generations. Thus the characters which appear in an immediate offspring are called "Dominant" and the other which are unexpressed and may be seen later are referred to as "Recessive".

Q8. What is "familital disorder or tendency" ?

Ans. Some of the disorders or disease are seen in families suggestive of inheritance however they lack conclusive evidence of genetic inheritance. These are referred as "familial disorders or tendencies".

Q9. Mention few examples of dominant inherited disorders of teeth ?

Ans. Hypoplasia of enamel, denitin dysplasia and dentinogenesis imperfecta.

Q10. What are the probable causes of congenital developmental anomalies ?

Ans. Various factors have been suggested as probable causes which result in congenital developmental anomalies. They are genetic, infections, physical injuries, hormones, nutritional, vascular interference, drugs chemicals, radiations, maternal diseases and defects in embryonic development.

Q11. What is agnathia ?

Ans. Agnathia is an extgremely rare condition wherein complete absence of either maxilla or mandible occurs.

Q12. What is micrognathia ?
Ans. Micrognathia is term used to describe small jaw bone. It could be either maxilla or mandible . Micrognathia of mandible is more common than maxilla.

Q13. Classify true micrognathia.
Ans. True micrognathia are either congenital or acquired. No definite etiological factors are known for congenital micrognathia. Whereas infection and trauma to the developing TMJ and jaw bones in postnatal period is believed to be the cause of qcquired type of micrognathia.

Q14. What is macrognathia ?
Ans. Increase in size of maxilla or mandible are referred to as macrognathia.

Q15. What are the causes of macrognathia ?
Ans. Hyperplasia of condyle, hyperpituitarism, and certain bone disorders like Paget's disease, leontosis ossea are the few conditions in which macrognathia is seen.

Q16. What is Facial hemihypertrophy ?
Ans. Gross asymmetry of two halves of face suggestive of increased length of one side in known as facial hemihypertrophy.

Q17. Mention the etiology of facial hemihypertrophy.
Ans. Define cause is unknown. However various factors like chromosomal abnormality, trauma, hormonal imbalance, localized alterations during intrauterine life, vascular abnormalities and lymphatic abnormalities are believed to be contributory to the abnormality.

Q18. Mention few oral manifestations of facial hemihypertrophy.
Ans. Teeth on affected side may show increase in crown and root size, and rate of development of teeth is accelerated. Either all or few teeth may be effected. Bone on effected size is large, wide and thicker. The bone may show increase thickness on trabeculae. Half of the tongue on

effected side appears enlarged with prominent lingual papillae. The mucosa may appear thick and velvety.

Q19. What is hemifacial atrophy ?
Ans. Hemifacial atrophy is progressive atrophy of one side of facial tissues.

Q20. Enumerate the etiology of hemifacial atrophy.
Ans. Even though definet etiological factor and pathogenesis is not known, certain factors are found to be associated with this progressive hemifacial atrophy. These suggested factors include trauma, infectin, genetical abnormality, trophic malfunction of the cervical sympathetic nervous system, and a form of scleroderma.

Q21. Mention the most universally acceptable classification If malocclusion.
Ans. The classification of Angle proposed in 1899 is the most acceptable classification for malocclusion. Malocclusion is broadly classified into three groups in this classification.

Q22. What is hypomaxilla ?
Ans. Hypomaxilla is defective formation of maxilla in its size. The small size maxilla may give appearance of depressed middle third of face, depressed nasal saddle and reduced height of face.

Q23. What is bossing ?
Ans. Prominent frontal bone eminences are known as bossing of frontal bone.

Q24. What is Vander Woude's syndrome ?
Ans. The association of congenital pits of lower lip with either cleft lip or cleft palate is known as Vander Woude's syndrome.

Q25. What are the developmental or congenital abnormalities of lips ?
Ans. Cleft lip, hare lip, pits of lip, commissural pits, double lip, and fistula of lip.

Q26. What are the findings of Ascher's syndrome ?
Ans. Ascher's syndrome is very rare. The findings consists of acquired double lip, blepharochalasis, and nontoxic thyroid enlargement.

Q27. What is blepharoachalasis ?
Ans. Blepharochalasis is drooping of the tissue between the eyebrow and the edge of eyelids, so that tissue hangs loosely over the eyelid.

Q28. Classify the cleft lip.
Ans. Cleft lip can be unilateral or bilateral in upper lip. Bilateral cleft lip is also known as harelip. The cleft lip can be either incomplete or complete with the involvement of nostril or palate.
In lower lip however it is mostly midline cleft lip.
Cleft lip of upper lip are more common than lower lip.

Q29. What are the causes of cleft palate ?
Ans. Many etiologic factors have been suggested. He redoty genetic is the most important factor among them.
The other factors include nutritional disturbances, administration of corticosteroids during pregnancy, riboflavin deficiency, Vitamin A (both hypo and hyper), stress, defective vascular supply to the area involved, and certain teratogenic drugs and chemicals.

Q30. What are the effects of cleft palate and lip?
Ans. Cleft palate and lip cause considerable psychological and physical effects. Psychological or mental trauma due to clinical evident facial defect is very significant. Physical and functional problems of clefts include difficulty in suckling, difficulty in eating, drinking, speech and malocclusion. Regurgitaion of fluids through the nose is a serious handicap.

Q31. What are the clinical manifestations of Peutz Jegher's syndrome ?

Ans. The Peutz Jegher's syndrome is hereditary intestinal polyposis syndrome, wherein intestinal polyposis, and orofacial pigmentation are the findings, Intestinal polyposis may cause frequent episodes of abdominal pain and signs of intestinal obstruction. There is strong tendency for development of malignancy in multiple polyposis of colon.

Q32. What is ephelides ?

Ans. Ephelides are small single or multiple melanotic nodules.

Q33. Give different names of Fordyce's disorder.

Ans. Fordyce's disorder is also known Fordyce spots, and Fordyce granules. Aggregation of these granules is also referred as sebaceous nevi.

Q34. What is sebaceous nevi ?

Ans. Aggregation of Fordyce granules are referred as sebaceous nevi. The Fordyce granules are ectopic sebaceous gland when may be located in labial and buccal mucosa.

Q35. Give the clinical appearance of Fordyce granules ?

Ans. Fordyce granules appear as yellowish or whitish spots on the mucosa. Aggregation or closely arranged Fordyce spots may appear as patch. They are usually bilateral in distribution.

Q36. Name the conditions which are considered in differential diagnosis of sebaceous nevi ?

Ans. Lichen planus, leukoplakia, linea alba buccalis, and candidiasis.

Q37. What is the etiology of Fordyce spots ?

Ans. The Fordyce spots or sebaceous nevi may occur due to inclusion of ectoderm having some of the potentialities of the skin into the oral mucosa during development.

Q38. Give the management of sebaceous nevi.
Ans. Sebaceous nevi or Fordyce granules are asymptomatic abnormality therefore do not require any treatment. However in individuals who are apprehensive of their malignant potentialities, an assurance and education on their benign nature may be required to allay the fear.

Q39. Name few developmental disorders of tongue.
Ans. Macroglossia, Microglossia, Ankyloglossia, Bifid tongue, Fissured tongue, and Median Rhomboid glossitis.

Q40. What is ankyloglassia ?
Ans. Ankyloglossia is term used to describe the condition resulting from short lingual frenum or absence of lingual frenum. The hsort frenum may be attached too close to tip of tongue. All these result in restricted movement of tongue. This condition is also tongue tie.

Q41. What is the etiology of macroglossia ?
Ans. Macroglossia or enlargement may be either congenital or secondary due to haemangioma, lymphangioma or due to deposition of amyloid. The secondary macroglossia may also be associated with hormonal disorders like hyperpituitarism or hypothyroidism (cretinism).

Q42. Write the clinical features of scrotal tongue ?
Ans. Scrotal tongue is developmental malformation presenting with deep fissures or cracks on the surface. There fissures are often radiating out from central longitudinal groove. The condition is often asymptomatic however stagnation of food and debris in deep fissure may cause pain or burning sensation.

Q43. Name one syndrome associated with scrotal tongue.
Ans. Melkersson Rosenthal syndrome in which fissured scrotal tongue, edema of lips and facial paralysis are associated findings.

Q44. What is Median Rhomboid Glossitis ?
Ans. Median Rhomboid Glossitis is a condition believ3ed to occur due to failure of the tuberculum impar to retract before fusion of two halves of tongue therefore it is a developmental anomaly of tongue. However its origin as a result of developmental anomaly has been disputed due to the fact that no cases of median Rhomboid glossitis was found in one study involving 10000 children. Recently candidial infection as one of the etiological factors has been suggested.

Q45. Give the clinical features of Median Rhomboid Glossitis.
Ans. Median Rhomboid glossitis appears clinically as an ovoid, diamond or rhomboid shaped reddish, depapillated area on the dorsal surface of the tongue immediately anterior to circumvallate papillae. It may appear as slightly raised area. It is more common in male than in females. The condition may be asymptomatic or sometimes may be painful.

Q46. What is aplasia ?
Ans. Congenital absence of salivary glands called aplasia.

Q47. What is atresia ?
Ans. Congenital absence or congenital occlusion of duct of any major salivary gland is called atresia.

Q48. Write the manifestations of ectodermal dysplasia.
Ans. Ectodermal dysplasia is also called hereditary hypohidrotic or anhidrotic ectodermal dysplasia. It is a hereditary condition characterized by congenital dysplasia of one or more structure of ectodermal origin or their appendages. The manifestations include hypohidrosis, hypotrichosis and hypodontia. Various abnormalities like dry skin, thin and sparse hair, andontia, absence of sweat glands, depressed nose, and pronounced supraorbital ridges and frontal bossing may be prominent features. The individuals suffer from hyperpyrexia due to absence of sweat glands.

Q49. What is the genodermatoses ?
Ans. Term genodermatoses is used to describe certain hereditary skin disorders which are accompanied by various systemic manifestations.

Q50. What is genokeratoses ?
Ans. Genokeratoses are the hereditary skin diseases associated with abnormal keratinization process.

Q51. Write the clinical manifestations of von Recklinghausen's syndrome.
Ans. The condition is multiple neurofibromatosis. It is inherited as an autosomal dominant condition. The syndrome manifests with simultaneous appearance of brown pigmentation of skin and multiple neurofibromatosis. These are nodular tumourous growth of peripheral nerves.

Q52. What is Gardner's syndrome ?
Ans. Garder's syndrome is a rare condition exhibiting multiple osteomas of jaw bones, dermoid and sebaceous cysts, associated with intestinal polyps and multiple impacted supernumerary teeth.

Q53. Write manifestations of Albright's syndrome.
Ans. The syndrome consisting of polyostiotic fibrous dysplasia of bone, brown pigmentations (Café au lait) of the skin, bony deformities and precocious sexual development is referred as Albright's syndrome.

Q54. In which year Cannon first described the condition of white sponge nevus ?
Ans. In 1935, Cannon described the condition of white folded, spongious appearance of oral mucosa. It is known as Cannon's disease or familial white folded dysplasia of oral mucosa or white sponge nevus.

Q55. Write the oral lesions of white sponge nevus.
Ans. Oral mucosal lesions may be congenital being present at birth or may develop later. The lesions cover a wide area of oral mucosa. These are white thick patches. The

thickened mucosa appears folded or corrugated. The white thickened areas may be present on the mucosa of cheek, lips, tongue, gingival and floor of oral cavity. They are usually bilateral.

Q56. Write the microscopic picture of white sponge nevus.
Ans. Microscopic picture in white sponge nevus is charactgerised by hyperkeratosis or hyperparakeratosis, and acanthosis. The cells of spinous layer show intracelluslar edema with pyknotic nuclei. In addition there may be evidence of parakeratin plugs running deep into prickle cell layer.

Q57. What are different developmental disorder of teeth?
Ans. Developmental disorders of teeth may be created to the size, shape, number, structure and eruption.

Q58. Classify the disorder of teeth effecting size.
Ans. The disorders involving size of teeth are broadly classified as microdontia and macrodontia. Again these are subdivided into true generalized, relative generalized and localised variations.

Q59. What is true generalized microdontia ?
Ans. In true generalized microdontia, all the teeth are smaller in size than normal.

Q60. What is relative generalized microdontia ?
Ans. The teeth are usually of normal size or slightly smaller, however the jaw bones are larger tham normal. Hence the teeth appear smaller even though they are of normal size. They are relatively smaller in size in comparison to the jaw bones.

Q61. Which are the teeth commonly effected by microdontia ?
Ans. Single tooth microdontia is very common condition. The most commonly effected teeth are maxillary lateral incisors

and maxillary third molars. The lateral incisor appear small and called "peg shaped" teeth. Crown is conical and tapering. The maxillary third molars also appear small, and malformed crown.

Q62. What is cause for true generalized macrodontia ?
Ans. True generalized macrodontia involving all the teeth, in which teeth are larger than in size, is a rare condition. The could be either hereditary or caused by pituitary gigantism.

Q63. What are the different disturbances associated with shape of teeth ?
Ans. The various conditions in which the shape of tooth or teeth is effected include germination, Fusion, Dense in dente, supernumerary cusps, pegshaped laterals, dens evaginatus, taurodontism, concrescence, dilacerations, hutchinoson teeth and supernumerary roots.

Q64. What is Gemination ?
Ans. Geminated teeth are anomalies which arise due to an attempt at a division of a single tooth by invagination, resulting in incomplete division of crown. The tooth may or may not appear larger, however the crown exhibits evidence of two cnopletely or partially separated crown. The root is usually is single with single root canal. The condition is not very common. It is more common in central or lateral incisors than other. The term "twinning" or "dichotomy" is used to describe the condition.

Q65. What is fusion of teeth?
Ans. Fusion of teeth is union of two separated tooth germs. The tooth germs may be of normal sequence or between are normal tooth gem with supernumerary tooth germ. Depending on the time at which the union has occurred, the fusion may be complete or incomplete. Clinically tooth appears large. If the fusion of tooth occurs after crown formation, the root may unite to form one root and one canal with two separate crowns. Fusion may occur in deciduous as well as in permanent dentition.

Q66. What is concrescence ?
Ans. Concrescence is a form of fusion of two neighboring teeth after completion of root formation. The roots unit by cementum.

Q67. What is dilaceration ?
Ans. The term dilaceratin refers to sharp bending of toothe either in root or crown. This is usually caused by trauma while tooth is being fourmed. The bend may occur anywhere along the length of tooth. Commonly it occurs in root.

Q68. What is clinical importance of diagnosis of dilacerated tooth ?
Ans. The dilacerated tooth appears normal clinically unless effected by caries or trauma. However the tooth may cause problem while extraction and for endodontic treatment.

Q69. What are the cuspal abnormalities ?
Ans. Cuspal abnormalities include accessory susp and more prominent cusp.

Q70. What is talon cusp ?
Ans. Talon cusp is projection arising from cingulum of incisors. It appears similar to an eagle's talon. The talon cusp may contain enamel, dentine and pulpal extension.

Q71. Mention the problems associated with the talon cusp.
Ans. Talon cusp may cause esthetic problems, occlusal interference, occlusal trauma, and increased incidence of carried around cusp. Endodontic treatment may also cause problems. Prophylactic resection of cusp may necessitate endodontic treatment for the tooth.

Q72. What is "Dens in Dente"?
Ans. "Dense in dente" is a developmental anomaly of tooth, modtly seen in anterior teeth. It is an invagination occurring on the lingual aspect of the tooth. The

invagination occurs as extension or deepening of lingual pit. The invagination may even invade root portion causing widening of root canal and root. The invaginated deep lingual pit is surrounded by enamel tissue. "Dens in dente" is also known as "dens invaginatus" or "tooth in tooth" or "pregnant tooth" or "invaginated odontome".

Q73. What is radicular variety of "Dens in dente" ?
Ans. Radicular variety of "Dens in dente" occurs due to invagination resulting from infolding of Hertwig's root sheath. The invagination occurs form apical end of root. The root appears bulky with wide opening.

Q74. What is clinical significance of "dens in dente" ?
Ans. The invagination or deep pit is prone for food impaction resulting in caries. In few instances the deep invagination may communicated with pulpal tissue making it accessible for infection. Periapical lesions like abscess are more often associated with such teeth.

Q75. What is "Dens Evaginatus" ?
Ans. "Dens evaginatus" is another developmental anomaly associated with shape of tooth. Clinically dens evaginatus appears as extra cusp or globule on the occlusal surface. It is not very common but the incidence is associated with premolars more often. It can occur on molars also.

Q76. What is clinical significance of "Dens evaginatus" ?
Ans. "Dens evaginatus" which is seen as prominent additional cusp like structure on occlusal surface may interfere with occlusion. The tooth is more prone for caries. Extra cusp may also interfere in proper eruption of tooth and may cause displacement of tooth.

Q77. What is taurodontism ?
Ans. Taurodontism is abnormality of tooth in which enlargement of crown occurs at the expense of root. The term "taurodontism" means bull like tooth. The crown appears wide and enlarged with short roots. It is more common

developmental disorder in molars than other teeth. Pulp chamber is very wide.

Q78. Mention types of taurodontism.
Ans. Taurodont may be divided into hypotaurodont, mesotaurodont and hypertaurodont. However this is not much significant except that hypertaturodontism is extreme from where in bifurcation or trifurcation may be located almost hear apices.

Q79. What are the radiological appearance of taurodont ?
Ans. Radiologically affected taurodont appears rectangular in shape rather than tapering cervically. The pulp chambers appears unusually wide and large. Roots appear small. Furcation of root may be more nearer to apical end.

Q80. What is the significance of accessory roots ?
Ans. The accessory roots may occur in association with any teeth. However the additional roots are most often seen in mandibular first molar and maxillary permanent third molar and maxillary permanent lateral incisor.

Q81. What are the different anomalies associated with number of teeth ?
Ans. The nabnomalies associated with number of teeth include anodontia, superuerary teeth, mesiodens, and paramolar etc.

Q82. What is oligodontia ?
Ans. Oligodontia is complete absence of teeth in jaw bones. IT is also called anodontia or hypodontia.

Q83. Classify anodontia.
Ans. Anodontia may be classified as true and false or acquired.

Q84. What is true anodontia ?
Ans. True anodontia or hypodontia is the condition where the teeth are not formed as there is failure of odontogenesis.

Q85. Classify true anodontia.
Ans. True anodontia may either be partial (single tooth) or total (all teeth).

Q86. Which teeth fail to form ?
Ans. In prtial anodonti, the maxillary permanent lateral incisors, third molars and mandibular permanent central incisors may be absent.

Q87. What is the significance of anodontia ?
Ans. Missing teeth may be part of a generalized syndrome like hereditary ectodermal dysplasia, hence examination of other parts or tissue become mandatory. The clinically missing teeth may be as a matter of fact be impacted. Therefore detailed clinical and radiological examination is essential to plan the treatment. Absence of permanent successor may permit the deciduous tooth to remain in arch for long period. Such retained deciduous teeth may be required to be retained by proper treatment.

Q88. What is false or acquired anodontia ?
Ans. Clinically missing teeth due to extraction for various pathological conditions or loss of teeth due to injury is called false or acquired anodontia. Clinically sound teeth may be required to be removed as part of orthodontics treatment planning.

Q89. What are the supernumerary teeth ?
Ans. The supernumerary teeth are extra teeth or additional teeth which are formed in addition to normal number. They my resemble in shape with neighboring tooth or may differ in shape completely. If the supernumerary tooth resembles normal tooth, this may be referred to as accessory tooth.

Q90. Mention the sites of occurrence of supernumerary teeth more often.
Ans. The supernumerary teeth occur more often in maxillary anterior teeth region and mandibular premolar region.

Q91. What are the names of supernumerary teeth found in different locations ?

Ans. Supernumerary teeth occurring between maxillary central incisors are referred as "mesiodens". Supernumerary teeth ccurring either buccally or lingually to molars are referred to as "paramolars". The rudimentary additional tooth occurring distal to third molar is sometimes referred as "fourth molar or distomolar".

Q92. Describe mesiodens ?

Ans. Mesiodens is the supernumerary tooth occurring between maxillary central incisors. The mesiodens may be single or multiple. These may erupt between the maxillary central incisors or may be found impacted and unerupted. Sometimes they are found in reverse direction in the maxilla.

Mesiodens are the most common of the supernumerary teeth.

Q93. Mention few conditions where multiple supernumerary teeth are found.

Ans. Multiple impacted supernumerary teeth are one of the findings of Garder's syndrome. The other findings include multiple osteomas, dermoid cysts and intestinal polyposis.

Multiple impacted supernumerary teeth are also occur in cleido cranial dysostosis or dysplasia.

Q94. What are the clinical features of cleido cranial dysplasia ?

Ans. Cleido cranial dysplasia is characterized by abnormalities of skull bones, teeth, jaws, clavicles and long bones.

Fontanelles of skull remain open for prolonged period. Skull bones are prominent and frontal bossing is evident. Clavicles are absent therefore individuals can bring the shoulder together or closer in forward position.

Maxilla is underdeveloped and paranasal sinuses are also small. High arched palate is a common feature.

The deciduous teeth remain retained for prolonged time. Unerupted succeeding teeth may remain in jaw bones.

There are many supernumerary teeth which remain impacted.

Q95. What is eruption sequestrum ?
Ans. During process of eruption, small spicules of bone overlying the occlusal surface of molar may get separated or sequestrated. These fragments get sequestracted through the overlying mucosa.

Q96. What are the predeciduous teeth ?
Ans. Predeciduous teeth are also called prenatal teeth. These are hornified., tiny structures which are present in mandibular incisor area. These are mobile and require removal.

Q97. What are the natal teeth ?
Ans. The deciduous teeth which erupt prematurely either at the time of birth or within few weeks are referred to as natal teeth. These are larger than prenatal teeth. Natal teeth may be required to be retained unlike prenatal which are extracted or removed.

Q98. What are submerged teeth ?
Ans. Teeth which are ankylosed to bone, do not erupt completely and remain below the occlusal plane. Deciduous molar teeth whose succeeding teeth are absent fail to erupt completely and remain at low level than neighbouring permanent teeth.

Q99. What are the types of abnormalities associated with structure of hard tissues of teeth ?
Ans. Hard tissues are formed in three stages. First the organic matrix is formed. The deficiency of matrix may lead to hypoplasia and excessive matrix formation leads to hyperplasia. During the second stage the mineral salts are deposited onto the matrix. This is called mineralization. Deficiency of mineralization will result in hypomineralisation or hypocacification. Third stage of hard tissue formation includes maturation, which involves

reorganization of mineral salts and removal of water. The defect in this stage may result in hypomaturation.

Q100. What are the clinical features of hypomineralised enamel ?

Ans. Hypomineralised enamel appears clinically soft. The amounf of enamel is normal but it is soft and lack strength. Therefore, quantity of enamel remains unaffected but quality is deficient.

Q101. What are the clinical features of hypoplasia of enamel ?

Ans. Hypoplasia is related to deficient amounf of organic matrix of enamel. Therefore amount of enamel deposited may be less or thin. The quality of enamel may remain unaltered even though amounf of enamel is less than normal. Hardness and strength of enamel remains unaltered.

Q102. Classify the disorders of enamel related to its structure.

Ans. The disorders of structure of enamel are classified as (a) hereditary and (b) environmental.

Q103. Mention the disorders manifesting enamel hypoplasia.

Ans. Enamel hypoplasia may be seen in Amelogenesis Imperfecta, and environmental enamel hypoplasia associated with local infection, trauma, congenital syphilis, hypocalemia, nutritional deficiency, exanthematous fever, ingestion of drugs like tetracycline and ingfestion of chemicals like fluoride.

Q104. What are the different names of Amelogenesis Imperfecta ?

Ans. Amelogenesis Imperfecta is also known as Hereditary enamel dysplasia, hereditary brown enamel and hereditary brown opalescent teeth.

Q105. What is Amelogenesis imperfecta ?
Ans.   Amelogenesis imperfecta represents a group of hereditary defects of enamel. It is further classified into different types based on clinical, histologic and genetic criteria. All the other tissues of teeth are not affected as amelogenesis imperfecta is entirely ectomermal disturbance.

Q106. What are the types of Amelogenesis Imperfecta ?
Ans.   Basing on clinical, histologic and genetic criteria, the amelogenesis Imperfecta is further gouped as hypoplastic, hypocalcified and hypomaturative.
Hypoplastic is mostly autosomal dominant and presents as pitted and rough areas and enamel is thin.

Q107. Give clinical features of Amelogenesis Imperfecta.
Ans.   Enamel in hypoplastic type appears thin but hard. The enamel is soft and can be chipped off in hypocalcified type. All the teeth may be effected to varying degree. The teeth may appear discolored from yellow to dard brown. Some parts of crown may exhibit chalky white hypoplastic areas. In severe form the enamel may be absent.

Q108. What are the exanthematous diseases which may cause enamel hypoplasia ?
Ans.   Exanthematous conditions like measles, chicken pox and scarlet fever during formative period of enamel may interfere with enamel formation. The hypoplasia in these types are of pitting surface type. Only few teeth are effected which generally are formative stage during first two years.

Q109. What is "mulberry molars" type of hypoplasia ?
Ans.   Hypoplasia occurring on molars due to congenital syphilis is referred to "Mulberry molar". The surface appears with multiple pits, loss of cusps, and narrowed occlusal plate. These molars are also referred as "Moon's molars" or "Fournier's molars".

Q110. What is turner's tooth ?
Ans.   This is a type of hypoplasia occurring in single teeth. It affects permanent teeth. Periapical infection of deciduous teeth may cause disturbance to calcification of underlying permanent successor, resulting in hypoplasia. This is referred to as Turner's hyhpoplasia. It mostly occurs in premolars or may be in maxillary permanent incisors.

Q111. What is mottled enamel ?
Ans.   Mottled enamel is a type of enamel hypoplasia associated with fluoride ingestion.

Q112. What is the safe level of fluoride in water ?
Ans.   Fluoride level in water below 0.9 to 1 pp, is considered as safe as there is no evidence of any hypoplastic changes.

Q113. What is the pathogenesis of fluoride related hypoplasia ?
Ans.   Exact mechanism of production of hypoplasia is not known. However it is believed that fluoride affects the ameloblasts and their function.

Q114. Mention the types of mottled enamel (fluorosis).
Ans.   Clinically the hypoplastic changes may vary from negligible to severely affected. These are (a) questionable changes where in occasional white spots are visible on surface of tooth (b) mild changes which are characterized by wide areas of opaque or white spots. (c) moderate changes are associated with pitting and brownish staining of surface and (d) servere form exhibiting deep and wider pitting, giving appearance of corroded teeth. These theeth affected by servere form tend to fracture or wear off at faster rate.

Q115. What is hereditary opalescent dentine ?
Ans.   Hereditary opalescent dentine is also called dentinogenesis imperfecta. It is a hereditary developmental disorder. Dentine formation is defective in this disorder.

Q116. which condition is usually associated with dentinogenesis imperfecta ?
Ans. Osteogenesis imperfecta is usually associated with dentinogenesis imperfecta.

Q117. Classify dentinogenesis imperfecta.
Ans. Shields and his co-workers have classified dentinogenesis imperfecta into three types.
Types I, the dentinogenesis imperfecta that always occurs in families with osteogenesis imperfecta.
In Type II the dentinogenesis imperfecta does not occur in association with osteogenesis imperfecta.
Type III is an autosomal dominant trait and is characterized by the clinical features of type I and II but also with multiple pult exposures in deciduous teeth.

Q118. Write the clinical features of dentinogenesis imperfecta.
Ans. Invariably deciduous teeth are more often affected than permanent teeth in type I whereas both the dentition may be affected in type II and type III. The color of teeth may vary grey to yellowish brown but they exhibit typical opalescent blue hue. Even though enamel is not affected but is lost due to chipping or fracture. This is explained on the basis of loss of scalloped attachment between enamel and dentin. Dentin becomes prone for more raid resorption. Hence the occlusal surface wear off and become flat.

Q119. Write radiological features of dentinogenesis Imperfecta.
Ans. Continued formation of dentine at faster rate is most prominent feature in type I and II. Therefore pulp chamber and canals are partially or totally oblit4erated. This obliteration of pulp chambers is seen in both deciduous and permanent as per the involvement. The roots are shorter. The other tissues of periodontium are unaffected.

In type III, the features are quite different. Pulp chamber and canals appear wider due to thin dentine, roots are shorter.

Q120. Write histological features of dentine of teeth in dentinogenesis Imperfecta.
Ans. Rate of deposition is very fast. Therefore the dentine deposited in type type I and II of Dentinogenesis Imperfecta is unorganized. Dentinal tubules are very wide and few in number. In some areas they are absent. Dentine may remain less calcified. Presence of osteodentine may be seen.

Q121. What is dentin dysplasia ?
Ans. Dentin dysplasia is a genetic disorder affecting the formation of dentine and roots. The roots are either short or absent. Therefore, it is referred to as "Rootless teeth".

Q122. What are the types of dentine dysplasia ?
Ans. Coronal and radicular types. Radicular type of abnormality more common than coronal tyupe of dentine dysplasia.

Q123. Write clinical and radiological features of coronal type of dentin dysplasia.
Ans. Both the dentitions may be affected. The color and appearance of teeth in general appear as in dentinogenesis imperfecta. Colour is dark ranging from grey to brown, yellow or opalescent blue. However the color changes may not be evident in permanent teeth. Radiologically obliteration of pulp chambers may be seen in deciduous teeth. However the permanent teeth exhibit abnormally large pulp chambers with foci of radiopacities suggestive of pulp stones.

Q124. Write clinical and radiological features of radicular type of dentin dysplasia.
Ans. In radicular type of dentine dysplasia, both the dentitins may be affected. The teeth clinically appear normal. However they exhibit extreme mobility and get exfoliated soon. Roots are either small or absent. Radiologically the

teeth exhibit obliteration of pulp chamber and canals. The typical feature is appearance of small circular radiolucencies resembling periapical cyst or granuloma in the apical ends of roots of teeth in this condition.

Q125. Write the histological features of dentine in dentine dysplasia.

Ans. In coronal type, the dentine deposited in tubular and amorphous in root portion. In coronal part it is more organized and resembles normal dentine. However in permanent teeth dentine is normal and multiple pulp stones are present in pulp.

In radicular type, the dentin is found obliterating pulp chamber. The dentin is found unorganized and consists of lumps of tubular dentine and osteodentin.

Q126. What is the deifference between dentinogenesis imperfecta and odontodysplasia ?

Ans. Dentinogenesis imperfecta is a condition of abnormality in dentine formation and odontodysplasia is a condition where in both enamel and dentine are affected.

Q127. What is odontodysplasia ?

Ans. Odontodysplasia is an unusual anomaly involving one or many teeth in one area. Maxillary teeth are the teeth which are involved more often, than mandibular. Anterior teeth have more probability of involvement than posterior. The affected teeth exhibit delay in eruption or remain unerupted. Their shape is irregular and distorted.

Q128. Write radiological teatures of odontodysplasia.

Ans. The tissues like enamel and dentine are hypocalcified. They exhibit less density and more radiolucency. Pulp chambers appear wider. As the teeth show marked reduction of opacity, the term "Ghost teeth" is used to describe the radiological appearance of unerupted affected teeth in odontodysplasia.

Q129. Describe the histological picture of teeth affected in odontodysplasia.

Ans. The most characteristic feature of these teeth are reduced amount of dentine, wider area of predentine, presence of large areas of interglobular dentine (hypocalcified). The enamel is less calcified.

Q130. What is the difference between embedded and impacted teeth ?
Ans. The embedded teeth are the teeth which fail to erupt due to lack of eruptive force. Whereas impacted are those prevented from erupting by some physical barrier in path of eruption.

Q131. Classify the classification of mandibular third molar ?
Ans. The impactions of mandibular third molar are classified into mesioangular, distoangular, horizontal, vertical and inverted. The impacted molars exhibit either buccal tilt or lingual tilt.

Q132. What are the complications of impacted mandibular third molars ?
Ans. Local or radiating pain, ear pain, headache, pain in temporal region, difficulty in mastication, food impaction, caries, proximal caries of adjacent tooth, malocclusion, pericoronitis, pericoronal abscess and submasetric or pterygomandibular space infection leading to trismus, are the few common complications. Other rare complications are developmet of dentigerous cyst, and osteomyelitis.

Q133. What are the different names of osteogenesis imperfecta?
Ans. Osteogenesis imperfecta is also known as "Brittle bone disease", Fragilitas ossium, osteopsathyrosis and Lobstein disease.

Q134. What is osteogenesis Imperfecta ?
Ans. Osteogenesis imperfecta is a serious diseases affecting mesodermal tissues. Multiple parts are affected in this disorders.

Q135. Give clinical manifestations of osteogenesis imperfecta.

Ans. The chief manifestations in osteogenesis imperfecta are seen in bones as increased fragility and porosity. The bones become prone for fracture. Multiple fractures in early life will lead to multiple deformities. Callus formation with or without fractures may occur. The individuals exhibit pale blue sclera. The sclera is thin and for this reason pigmented choroids is visible through appearing light blue.

Teeth abnormalities similar to dentinogenesis imperfecta may be present.

Q136. Mention the conditions in which blue sclera is present.

Ans. There are various abnormal condition, in which blue sclera is a common feature. Even in normal individuals as well the blue sclera may be present. The ebnormal conditions inlucde osteogenesis imperfecta, osteopetrosis, Marfan's syndrome, fetal rickets, and Ehlers Danlos syndrome.

Q137. What is Caffey's disease ?

Ans. Infantile cortical hyperostosis is originally described by Caffey and Silverman. Hence it is known as Caffey's disease or Caffey Silverman syndrome. This disease is characterized by unusual thickening of cortical plates.

Q138. Describe the general and oral manifestations of infactile cortical hyperostosis.

Ans. General manifestations of infantile cortical hyperostosis include tender, deeply placed soft tissue swellings, cortical thickening of various bones. Mandible is also affected giving rise to facial swelling. It is the most often affected bone. Clavicles are also affected. The secondary manifestations include paralysis, dysphagia, hyperirritability, anemia, and leukocytosis. However these are very common.

Q139. Write characteristic features of Marfan syndrome ?
Ans. Marfan syndrome is an autosomal dominant type hereditary disorder. The characteristic features of the disorder include excessive length of tubular bones resulting in long thin extremilites and spider like fingers. Other features include hyper extensibility of joints. The oral manifestations include high arched palate, bifid uvula ad malocclusion.

Q140. One famous personality was affected by marfan syndrome. Name the famous personality.
Ans. Abraham Lincoln, Former president of United States of America.

Q141. What is Down Syndrome ?
Ans. Down syndrome is disorder resulting from Trisomy 21. It is also called Mongolism.

Q142. What is Tridomy 21 ?
Ans. Presence of extra chromosome no 21 resulting in total of 47 chromosomes. The extra chromosome results in Down syndrome.

Q143. Write clinical features of Down syndrome ?
Ans. Patients affected by Down syndrome exhibit unbnormal mentality, flat face, large anterior fontanel, small slanting and oblique eyes. Overe all development is affected and is underdeveloped. Macroglossia with deep fissures is a common finding.

Q144. What is osteopetrosis ?
Ans. Osteopetrosis is an uncommon disease of bones and is also known as marble bone disease. It is an inherited disease.

Q145. Mention types of osteopetrosis.
Ans. There are two types, one is benign dominantly inherited form and second one is malignnt recessively inherited form.

Q146. Describe the clinical features of benign type of osteopetrosis.

Ans. It is a less severe form. It develops later in life. Therefore survival rate is good. This mild form of disease may be asymptomatic but for the occurrence of pathological fractures of various bones including mandible. Development of osteomyelitis at extraction socket site or at fracture site is common complication of osteopetrosis. Sclerosis of bone is predominant feature.

Q147. Write clinical feature of malignant type of osteopetrosis.

Ans. It is more severe and fatal form. It is either present at birth or occur in early period of life. Some affected are stillborn or die early soon after birth. Multiple bones are involved in development of sclerosis. The sclerosis of bones and nerve canals may lead to neurological disorders including optic nerve atroply facial palsy and loss of hearing etc. Pathological fractures and secondary infections are common. Fatality is usually associated with either severe anemia or severe secondary infection.

Q148. Describe the radiological findings of soteopetrosis.

Ans. Radiological picture varies depending on the extent of involvement of bones. However characteristic features of classic case of osteopetrosis, include diffuse, homogeneous, and symmetrical sclerotic changes with loss of bone marrow spaces. The cortical plates of bones appear thickened.

Q149. What is Rendu Osler weber syndrome ?

Ans. Rendu Osler weber disease is also referred to as Hereditary haemorrhagic telangiectasia ame conspicuous later in life. The lesions are characterized by spider like telangiectases. There are found commonly on face, neck, and chest. Intraorally the oral mucosa of tongue, buccal mucosa and gingival may be involved.

Q150. name the conditions considered for differential diagnosis of disease characterized by telangiectatic lesions.

Ans. There are innumerable conditions which exhibit telangiectatic skin and mucosal lesions. They are hereditary haemorrahagic telangiectasia, Sturge Weber disease, scleroderma, CREST syndrome and lupus erythematosus.

Q152. What are the bleeding and clotting times ins hereditary haemorrhagic telangiectasia ?

Ans. Both bleeding and clotting times are found normal.

Q153. Describe the clinical features of encephalotrigeminal angiomatosis.

Ans. It is a congenital but uncommon disorder characterized by angiomatosis and intracranial involvement. The typical skin angiomas are present on face, along with the distribution of trigeminal nerve. The other features are related to intracranial calcifications. Ocular involvement includeglaucoma, exophthalmos, and angioma of choroids.

Q154. What are tori ?

Ans. Tori are the bony protruburances present either on palate or mandible.

Q155. What is the etiology of tori ?

Ans. Even though various theories have been suggested, the hereditary cause seems to be more predominant in causation of tori.

Q156. Describe the torus palatinus.

Ans. Torus palatinus is slow growing protruburous growth in the midline of hard palate. The growth may be single or multiple. They are of different shapes including flat, nodular and spindle. Mucosa covering the tori may appear normal or blanched. The patients experience difficulty in speech and swallowing.

Q157. Describe the torus mandibularis.
Ans.   Torus mandibularis is invariably biteral. The protruburous growth occur on inner aspect of body of mandible in premolar region above mylohyoid ridge. It may occur on one side in few occasions. The size and shape vary considerably.

Q158. What is congenital epulis of new born ?
Ans.   Congenital epulis of new born, as name suggests, is seen at the time of birth and is present either on maxilla or mandible. It is nore common on maxilla. This epulis is pedunculated growth. The epulis may be of few millimeters to several centimeters. It is pink or dark pink in color. It exhibits smooth surface.

Q159. What are the Epstein's pearls ?
Ans.   Tiny white appearing cysts of palate described by Esptein in 1880 are known as Epstein pears. These occur from entrapped epithelial remnants along the midline.

Q160. What are the Bohn's nodules ?
Ans.   Bohn's nodules are also similar tiny cysts located on the posterior part of palate. They are present posteriorly at the junction of hard and soft palate. They are believed to derive from epithelial remnants of developing palatal minor salivary glands.

Q161. What are the fissural cysts ?
Ans.   The cysts arising from the epithelial remnants at the union of two embryonic processes are called fissural or inclusion cysts.

Q162. Name few fissural cysts occurring in orofacial region.
Ans.   These cysts may occur in either soft tissue alone or within bone. The cysts of soft tissue include nasoalveolar, thyroglossal cysts, dermoid cyst, Epstein pears and Bohn's nodules.

The bony cysts include median palatal, median anterior maxillary cysts, globulomaxillary and median mandibular cysts.

Q163. What is the location of globulomaxillary cysts ?
Ans. It is located in maxilla etween lateral and canine teeth. This is the location of union of globular and maxillary processes. However very few authors presently believe that there is no definite fusion between these two process, therefore chances of entrapment of epithelium is remote. Hence they believe that the globulomaxillary cyst may also be of odontogenic orifin instead of true fissural cyst.

Q164. What is the radiological picture of globulomaxillary cysts ?
Ans. Globulomaxillary cysts appears as inverted pear shaped well defined radiolucency between the roots of maxillary permanent lateral incisor and canine teeth. The causes divergence of roots.

Q165. What is the differential diagnosis of globulomaxillary cyst shadow in radiographs ?
Ans. Lateral periodontal cysts, apical periodontal cyst and odontogenic keratocysts may be considered in differential diagnosis in radiological picture of radiolucency between maxillary lateral incisors and canine.

Q166. What is nasoalveolar cyst ?
Ans. Nasoalveolar cyst is a rare inclusion cyst located in soft tissue and is believed to occur at the location of union of globular, lateral nasal process and maxillary process. It is also called nasolabial cyst.

Q167. Describe the clinical features of nasoalveolar cyst.
Ans. Nasoalveolar or nasolabial cyst may cause swelling in the mucobuccal fold and may be in the floor of nose also. It is usually asymptomatic except for asymmetry of face. It may cause some erosion of labial surface of maxilla due to pressure. It usually is not visible in radiographs.

Q168. What is the location of thyroglossal tract cyst ?
Ans. Thyroglossal duct or tract cyst may be located anywhere along the embryonic thyroglossal duct between foramen caecum of tongue and thyroid glands.

Q169. What is the origin of the thyroglossal duct cyst ?
Ans. The thyroglossal duct cyst arises from the cell remnants of the thyroglossal tract. The formation of cyst may be triggered by chronic infection or trauma.

Q170. Describe the clinical feature of thyroglossal tract cyst.
Ans. It is an uncommon cyst which is seen as a swelling in midline of neck and is usually asymptomatic. It may cause dysphagia if it is located high in the tract. It may lie in tongue near foramen caecum causing enlargement of tongue, which may cause difficulty in swallowing process.

Q171. What is the histologic picture of thyroglossal tract cyst ?
Ans. The thyroglossal tract cyst may be lined by either stratified squamous epithelium or ciliated columnar epithelium or intermediate transition type. The connective tissue wall may contain sometimes lymphoid and thyroid tissue also.

Q172. What is dermoid cyst ?
Ans. It is a form of cystic teratoma arising from embryonic epithelium. These cysts are believed to arise from entrapped multipotent epithelial debris in the midline during closure of mandibular and hyoid branchial arches. Hence the cyst may contain non epithelial structures as well.

Q173. Describe the clinical features of dermoid cyst.
Ans. The dermoid cyst occurring in the floor of the mouth is initially asymptomatic and small swelling located in floor of mouth. The large swellings may cause interference in mastication and swallowing processes. The cysts located in deeper structure may be visible as extra oral swelling in

submental area. The consistency varies from soft to firm commonly described as "doughlike" feeling.

Q174. What is the differential diagnosis of dermoid cyst ?
Ans. In differential diagnosis of dermoid cysts, the other considered are ranula, thyroglossal tract cyst, cystic hygroma and benign and malignant tumors of floor of mouth.

Q175. What is the thistological picture of dermoid cyst?
Ans. Histologically, the dermoid cyst presents a varied picture depending on the stage. It may present as epithelial lined cavity surroiunded by varied connective tissue. It may also contain kerating. On other occasion, one may find other structures like sebaceous glands, and hair follicles. The extreme cases may contain other tissues like bony and muscle tissue.

Q176. What are the causes of generalized intrinsic stains of teeth ?
Ans. Various etiological factors are believed to cause generalized staining of teeth. These include tetracycline stains, Amelogenesis imperfecta, Dentinogenesis imperfecta, fluorosis, Erythoblastosis fetalis and porphyria.

Q177. What is cherubism ?
Ans. Cherubism is an uncommon disease presenting as bilateral involvement of mandible. It is believed to be inherited disorder. It is characterized by multilocular cystic lesions on both sides of mandible. The word "cherubism" is given due to rounded appearance of face as there is bilateral symmetrical swelling. Even though mandible is commonly affected bone, maxilla may also be involved.

Q178. What is the status of dentition in cherubism ?
Ans. There may be premature shedding of deciduous teeth. Development and eruption of permanent teeth is affected, resulting in either absence or impaction of teeth.

Q179. How to differentiate intrinsic stains caused by tetracycline and porphyria ?

Ans. Tetracycline affected teeth exhibit yellow or orange fluorescence underultraviolet light, whereas the discolored teeth associated with porphyreia exhibit red fluorescence under ultraviolet rays.

Q180. Mention the clinical differential diagnosis of mid palatine cyst ?

Ans. Mid palatine cyst presents as swelling on the palate, posterior to incisive papilla. The other conditions which need consideration of differentiation are torus palatinus, adenoma, adenocarcinoma, and palatal abscess.

4.

INFECTIONS

Q1. What are the various agents which cause infections of orofacial tissues ?
Ans. Bacteria, spirochetes, fungi, viruses and parasites usually cause infections of orofacial tissues.

Q2. What is nonspecific infection ?
Ans. The infections of orofacial tissues which are caused by a broad group of microorganism is referred to as nonspecific infection.

Q3. What is specific infection ?
Ans. Specific infection is caused by specific organism like mycobacterium tuberculosis and corynebacteruim diphtheria, etc.

Q4. What are the infections which are characterized by white or yellow pseudomembrance?
Ans. Pseudomembrane may be seen in diphtheria, acute necrotizing ulcerative gingivitis, candidiasis and secondary syphilis.

Q5. What is stomatitis scarlatina ?
Ans. Oral mucosal manifestation of scarlet fever is stomatitis scarlatina. The mucosa may appear congested and inflamed. The throat mucosa appears fiery red and edema of faucial pillars.

Q6. Described the tongue lesions seen in scarlet fever.
Ans. Early in the course of dises the dorsum of toungue is coated with white coating and fungiform papilla which are edematous and hyperemic, appear as small red circular areas in white coating. This is described as strawberry

tongue. Later as the disease progresses, the shite coating is lost. The tongue appears deep red, and smooth with disappearance of filiform papilla. The hyperemic fungiform still persists. This appearance of tongue is described as raspberry tongue.

Q7. What are the factors which influence the initiation and severity of infections ?
Ans. Even though many infectins are caused by pathogenic microorganisms, some infections are caused by commensals. The factor which influence the infections are general health, immunity, nutritional status, hormonal imbalance, lowered resistance, and certain drugs or chemicals which disturb the normal microbial flora.

Q8. Which organism causes diphtheria ?
Ans. Diphtheria is an acute contagious disease caused by gram positive bacteria corynebacterium diphtheria.

Q9. What is the incubation period in diphtheria ?
Ans. The incubation period is 4 to 7 days in diphtheria. Then constitutional symptoms like malasise, fever, headache, and occasional vomiting may occur, followed by severe pharyngitis. Regional lymphadenitis may be seen.

Q10. What are the oral manifestations in diphtheria ?
Ans. Characteristic feature of the diphtheria in oral cavity is development of grayish or whitish pseudomembrane over the surface of tonsil, uvula, larynx, pharynx and gingival. The most common site is posterior part of oral cavity. This membrance consists of exudates dead cells, leukocystes and bacteria. The membrace is gelatinous and adherent over a ulcerated surface of mucosa. It leaves bleeding and ulcerated surface when peeled off.

Q11. What are the complications of diphtheria ?
Ans. As the disease progresses it may cause paralysis of soft palate resulting in regurgitation of liquids during drinking and these patients develop a peculiar nasal twang. Later it may involve the larynx resulting in edema of larynx and

mechanical blocking of larynx by pseudomembrane causeing suffocation, if the airway is not cleared. Other complications arise in cardiovascular and nervous systems as a result of toxemia. Both myocarditis and polyneuritis may devlop.

Q12. What is the management of diphtheria ?
Ans. The disease is treated by administration of antitoxins, and antibodies. The pseudomembrane shall be removed.
The disease may be prevented by prophylactic active immunization with diphtherja toxoid.

Q13. Which bacteria causes tuberculosis ?
Ans. Tuberculosis is an infectious granulomatous disease caused by acid fast bacillus mycobacterium tuberculosis.

Q14. What are the other granulomatous disorders ?
Ans. Granulomatous disorders other than tuberculosis are syphilis, sarcoidosis, actinomycosis, hostiocytosis X, Crohn's disease, foreign body granuloma and giant cell granuloma.

Q15. Mention the bacterial infections affecting the oral mucosa.
Ans. Oral mucosa may be affected by nonspecific mixed coccal infection, streptococcal hemolytic type, diphtheria, tuberculosis, syphilis, actinomycosis, Vincent's infection and leprosy.

Q16. What are different forms of tuberculosis ?
Ans. Tuberculosis may affect local tissues, or systems like respiratory systems (pulmonary), gastrointestinal tract, bones, lymphnode (scrofula), skin (lupus vulgaris) and it may disseminate through system causing wide spread manifestations. This is called military tuberculosis.

Q17. What are the oral manifestations of tuberculosis ?
Ans. Oral manifestation in tuberculosis are relatively uncommon. Among the oral soft tissues, the tougue is affected more often, followed by palate, lips, buccal

mucosa and gingival. The lesion may be nodular but most often is represented by irregular ulcer. The ulcer is painful. The ulcer tend to increase in size and is characterized by under mining margins. Rarely tuberculosis of gingival may occur which is characterized by diffuse byperemic, nodular or papillary proliferation of gingival tissue. Tuberculosis may also affect mandible and maxilla.

Q18. Describe the histologic picture to tuberculosis lesion.
Ans. The tuberculosis lesion exhibit foci of caseous nocrosis surrounded by epitheloid cells, lymphocytes and multinucleated giant cells. The mycobacterium tuberculosis may be present in these lesions.

Q19. Which disease resembles closely with tuberculosis lesion microscopically ?
Ans. Histological appearance of lesions of sarcoid resembles the lesions found in tuberculosis.

Q20. How to differentiate microscopically between tuberculosis and sarcoid lesion ?
Ans. Central caseation is absent in sarcoid lesion. The mycobacterium tuberculosis are also not isolated from these lesions, whereas these are positive findings of tuberculosis lesion.

Q21. What is cold abscess ?
Ans. As the name suggests, this absecess is cold and nonreacting in nature. It does not exhibit, produce hot and painful and inflammatory signs like induration and tenderness. However, the abscess may open up discharging the pus. Cold abscess is almost always a sequel to tubercular infection, anywhere in body. However, it is commonly associated with tuberculosis of lymph nodes or bones.

Q22. What is Herxheimer reaction ?
Ans. Herxheimer reaction is a altered reaction to antibiotic in chronic diseases. For example gummatous lesions of

tertiary syphilis causes sudden necrosis and destruction of tissue leading to perforation following vigorous course of antibiotics.

Q23. Is actionomycosis classified as fungus or bacteria ?
Ans. Even though in earlier period, the actinomycosis was considered to be a gungus. However, presently it is considered as bacteria. The term mycosis is misleading. The organisms behave serologically and biochemically as bacteria.

Q24. Which form of actinomycosis cause disease in human beings ?
Ans. Most often isolated organism is actinomycosis israelli.

Q25. What are the characteristic features of actinomycosis israelli ?
Ans. The organism are anaerobic, gram positive, non acid fast, and branched filamentous organism.

Q26. Classify actinomycosis disease.
Ans. Actinomycosis is classified anatomically depending on the tissue involvement. There are three forms. They are (1) cervicofacial (2) Abdominal and (3) Pulmonary forms.

Q27. Describe the cervicofacial actinomycosis.
Ans. Cervicofacial region is relatively most common of the three forms. The organism may enter the tissues through oral mucosa or skin. It may spread to neighbouring areas to involve bone, soft tissues, and salivary glands producing swelling and induration of the tissues. These swellings develop into abscesses which open on the skin surface discharging us containing typical "Sulfur Granules". It is a chronic condition. As the old sinuses tend to heal, new abscesses and sinuses form. Thus a patient over a period of time may exhibit a great deal of scarring disfigurement of facial and neck region. Bony involvement may cause specific type of osteomyelitis.

Q28. What are the sulfur granules ?
Ans. Sulfur granules are made up to colonies of organisms. These appear as yellow grains in pus.

Q29. What is the bistologic picture of actinomycosis ?
Ans. Typical lesion of actinomycosis presents a characteristic granulomatous one showing central abscess formation. The pus contains colonies of organisms.

Q30. What is the microscopic picture of sulfur granule ?
Ans. The colonies may appear as round and made up of a mesh work of filments. These filaments stain with haematoxylin but the peripheral club shaped ends of filaments stain eosinophilic. This typical appearance of radiating filaments is the basis for oftenly used term "Ray fungus".

Q31. What is the other name of syphilis ?
Ans. Syphilis is also referred to as Lues.

Q32. Which factor has reduced the incidence of centuries old disease syphilis ?
Ans. Advent of antibiotic like penicillin and tetracyclines has considerably lowered the incidence of syphilis.

Q33. What is the causative organism of syphilis ?
Ans. Syphilis is caused by infection with a spirochete Treponema pallidum.

Q34. Classify syphilis.
Ans. Syphilis is classified as (1) Acquired and (2) Congenital.

Q35. What is congenital syphilis ?
Ans. Congenital syphilis is development of abnormalities in developing structures during intrauterine period due to syphilitic infection in mother. In true sense, it is misnomer as the congenital syphilis is acquired from mother and manifestations are seen in offspring.

Q36. What is acquired syphilis ?

Ans. Acquired syphilis is infection by Treponema pallidum due to direct contact. IT manifests in different stages.

Q37. What are the different stages of acquired syphilis ?
Ans. Acquired syphilis manifests in different forms, if it is left untreated. The initial stage is primary stage, then secondary stage and later severe destructive tertiary stage.

Q38. What are the manifestations of primary stage of syphilis ?
Ans. The lesion in primary stage develops at the site of inoculation of organism. The incubation period is about 3 weeks after the contact of infection. The primary lesion is known as chancre. It is seen mostly in sexual organs. However, it may occur on lips and tongue as well. This primary lesion is in the form of elevated nodule with ulceration. The margins of ulcers show sharp, deep margins referred to as punched out ulcers. The ulcer is usually painless, however, pain may be present if secondary infection supervenes. Regional lymphadenitis is present. The organisms are found plenty in chancres.

Q39. Which are the infective stages of syphilis ?
Ans. Primary stage (Chancre) and secondary stage (mucous patches) are the most infective stages as the organism are found in plenty.

Q40. Which is the best method of demonstration of Treponema pallidum ?
Ans. Treponema pallidum stains poorly except by silver impregnation. Therefore, it can be best demonstrated by dark field microscope.

Q41. Which other organism is found to be similar to Treponema pallidum ?
Ans. Treponema pallidum like organisms may also be demonstrated in saliva of nonsyphilitic patients as another spirochete Treponema microdentium is present in saliva of

most of normal persons as well. This may be confused with spirochete Treponema pallidum.

Q42. Which of the lesions contain spirochetes Treponema pallidum ?
Ans. The spirochetes Treponema pallidum can be isolated from chance of primary stage, mucous patches of secondary stage and lymphnodes draining the chancre.

Q43. What is the differential diagnosis of chancre of lip ?
Ans. Chancre of lip shall be differentiated from traumatic ulcer, squamous cell carcinoma, cheilitis granulomatosa and drythema multiform.

Q44. What is the duration of chancre ?
Ans. Chancre may remain for few weeks in patients who do not receive treatment. The ulcer exhibits spontaneous healing within three weeks to four weeks.

Q45. What are the manifestations of secondary stage of syphilis ?
Ans. Primary lesion heals spontaneously within three weeks to four weeks. Then the affected person develops certain sessions of secondary stage in six to seven weeks after primary lesion. The manifestations of secondary stage include appearance of popular eruptions, on the skin and mucosa and mucous patches on oral mucosa.

Q46. What are the mucous patches ?
Ans. Oral mucosal lesions of secondary stage of syphilis are referred to as mucous patches. These are characterized by multiple, painless, grayish white plaques overlying an ulcerated surface. They are irregular in shape and most often occur on buccal mucosa, tongue and giniva. These areas are surrounded by erythematous zones.

Q47. What are the chances of infection from mucous patches ?
Ans. Mucous patches of secondary syphilis are higly infective as they contain numerous microorganisms.

Q48. What is the usual duration of secondary stage ?
Ans. Manifestations of secondary stage of syphilis heal spontaneously within few weeks, however, these do continue to keep on recurring for several years, till development of late stage manifestations (tertiary stage).

Q49. What are the manifestationso f tertiary stage of syphilis ?
Ans. Tertiary stage also referred to as late stage, develops as severe, destructive stage involving multiple organs and systems. It involves cardiovascular system, nervous system and various organs including facial bones. The lesions of tertiary stage of syphilis are non infective. Interstitial glossitis is also seen.

Q50. What is the localised lesion of tertiary stage of syphilis ?
Ans. Gumma is the main localised lesion seen in the tertiary syphilis.

Q51. Name the various locations of gumma ?
Ans. Gumma occurs most frequently on skin, mucous membrane, testes, liver, bones and tongue.

Q52. What is gumma ?
Ans. Gumma is a localised lesion of tertiary syphilis. It consists of a focal, granulomatous inflammatory mass with central necrosis. The size may vary from few millimeters to few centimeters.

Q53. Describe a gumma of oral tissue.
Ans. Intraorally the gumma may occur on tongue and palate. The gumma appears as nodular mass which may subsequently ulcerate. The gumma on palate causes perforation of palate by sloughing. The perforation follows vigorous antibiotic therapy (Herxheimer reaction).

Q54. What is Leutic glossitis ?
Ans. Leutic glossitis is interstitial or atrophic glossitis seen in tertiary syphilis. It is characterized by shrunken, smooth, depapillated and pale tongue.

Q55. What are the manifestations of congenital syphilis ?
Ans. Congenital syphilis is charcterised by variety of manifestations which occur in offsprings born to infected mother. The manifestations include bossing of frontal bones, hypomaxilla, low nasal bridge, high palatal arch, thickening of sternoclavicular end of clavicle, protruberance of mandible, rhagades, saber shin, abnormality in teeth, eighthnerve deafness and interstitial keratitis.

Q56. What are the oral manifestations of congenital syphilis ?
Ans. Rhagades, high palatal arch, hypomaxilla, protruded mandible, and hypoplasia of molars and incisors are the manifestations of congenital syphilis.

Q57. What is mulberry molar ?
Ans. Mulberry molar is a hypoplastic permanent first molar. The hypoplasia is caused by disturbance during development. The cusps and occlusal surface exhibits pitted hypoplasia, with shortening and narrowing of occlusal surface. The mulberry molar is one of the manifestations occurring in congenital syphilis. The fact that the first molar is effected in congenital syphilis, indicates that the development and initial calcification of first molar commence in intrauterine life only.

Q58. Which are the other teeth affectd in congential syphilis ?
Ans. Maxillary permanent central and lateral incisors are affected. Middle lobe is not developed hence, mesiodistal width of incisal third is less giving the appearance of the tooth which is described as "screw driver" incisor. Due to failure of development of middle lobe, may result in notching in middle of incisal edge. Lateral incisor may present as peg shaped.

Q59. What is "Hutchinson's triad" ?
Ans. Hutchinson triad include hypoplasia of teeth, eighth nerve deafness and interstitial keratitis.

Q60. What are rhagades ?
Ans. Rhagades are the development of radiating fissures around the opening of mouth. These are one of the various manifestations of congenital syphilis.

Q61. What are the investigations for syphilis ?
Ans. The investigation for syphilis include microbial examination and serological tests.

Q62. What are the different procedures for demonstration of Treponema Pallidum ?
Ans. The spirochete Treponema pallidum cannot readily be cultured. The organisms isolated from the lesions are identified and demonstrated by dark field microscopy. These spirochetes are motile. Hence, they are easily distinguished when they refract light in an otherwise dark microscopic field.
The Treponema pallidum can now be identified with fluorescent labeling techniques by use of specific syphilitic antiserum.

Q63. What serologic test are done for syphilis ?
Ans. The various serologic tests for syphilis include VDRL, Wassermann, complement fixation tests, kahn and kline test, flocculation tests, Trepenoma pallidum immobilization

(TPI) and fluorescent treponemal antibody aborption tests (FTA ABS).

Q64. Do the serological tests help in diagnosis of primary stage of syphilis ?
Ans. Not always. The serological tests may be negative in initial stages of primary lesions of syphilis. Isolation and identification of organism from the lesion and affected lymph node may be more diagnostic value in primary stage.

Q65. In which stages of syphilis, the serologic tests are found positive and useful ?
Ans. The serologic tests are found positive and useful in secondary and tertiary stages.

Q66. In which forms of syphilis the serologic tests are negative ?
Ans. The serologic tests may be negative in initial stages of primary infection and in persons affected by congenital syphilitic manifestations.

Q67. What is the treatment of syphilis ?
Ans. Antibiotics like penicillin is more effective. Procaine penicillin, penicillin in aluminium monostereate, or long acting penicillin are effective in management of syphilis.

Q68. What are the Donovan bodies ?
Ans. Donovan bodies are characteristic findings of biopsies in granuloma inguinale. These bodies are tiny elongated basophilic rods present within intracytoplasmic cysts in mononuclear phagocytes. These large mononuclear phagocyte are pathognomic of granuloma inguinale.

Q69. What are the differne names of acute necrotizing ulcerative gingivitis (ANUG) ?
Ans. Acute necrotizing ulcerative gingivitis is not and uncommon disease and is referred with various names. Vincent's gingivitis, Trench mouth, acute

ulceromembranous gingivitis, phagedenic gingivitis and fusospirochetal gingivitis are the other names.

Q70. Mention the types of vincent's gingivitis ?
Ans. Two recognized entities of vincent's gingivitis or acute necrotizing ulcerative gingivitis are well documented. They are (1) Acute and (2) Subacute form.

Q71. What is the causative agent of ANUG ?
Ans. It is caused by fusiform bacillus and a spirochete Borrelia Vincenti.

Q72. What are the predisposing factors in development of ANUG ?
Ans. In addition to causative agents, there are certain local and systemic factors which predispose to the disorder. The local factors include poor oral hygiene, smoking and trauma. The systemic factors include lowered resistance, vitamin C deficiency and vitamin B complex.

Q73. What is trench mouth ?
Ans. ANUG is also referred to as Trench mouth as the disease was found more prevalent among the toops in trenches during war times.

Q74. Describe the clinical features of ANUG ?
Ans. Acute necrotizing ulcerative gingivitis is manifested as local gingivitis affecting mostly papillary and marginal gingival. It may occur in any age but more common in young. The disease starts as severe gingivitis and bleeding gums. The punched out erosions or ulcers occur initially at papillary gingival and spreads to marginal gingival. The ulcerated or eroded area is covered by grayish, whitish pseudomembrane. The lesions may start in pericoronal flaps over erupting last molars and anterior teeth regions. Later it may spread to other areas. Bleeding from gingival is very spontaneous. Patients complain of metallic taste. Foetid odour is characteristic unpleasant finding. The systemic manifestations include fever and malaise.

Regional lymphadenitis is present. Excessive salivation is common feature.

Q75. What are the features of fusiform bacillus ?
Ans. The fusiform bacillus associated with ANUG is an elongated rod with tapered ends measuring 5 to 14 microns in length and 0.5 to 1.0 microns in diameters. This is non motile and weak gram positive and anaerobic organism.

Q76. Describe Borrelia Vincenti ?
Ans. Borrelia Vincenti is gram negative spirochete with three to six long spirals. It is motile and measures 10 to 15 microns in length. It is also anaerobic spirochete.

Q77. How do you manage ANUG ?
Ans. The management of ANUG include local and systemic. Local from of management include debridement and local use of oxygen liberating mouth washes. Later scaling and polishing can be under taken when acute phase subsides.
They systemic form of management include administration of antibiotics like penicillin or tetracycline. Specific antimicrobial agent like metronidazole which is most effective in anaerobic organisms can be given.
Metronidazole is given in dose of 200 to 400 mg tablets three times a day.

Q78. What is Cancrum Oris ?
Ans. Cancrum oris or Noma is a rapidly spreading gangrene of orofacial structures. It may result as a complication of ANUG, in a debilitating malnourished individuals. Seen mostly in children suffering with severe malnourishment specially hypoproteinemia. Vicents' organisms are associated with Noma or gangremous stomatitis.

Q79. Describe the clinical features of Noma.
Ans. Gangrenous stomatitis or Noma starts as small necrotic ulcer on gingival and rapidly spreads to adjacent tissues or tissues in contact with the surface of ulcer like buccal mucosa, and lips. The ulcerative lesion enlarges to become rapidly destructive and necrotic slough and loss of tissues.

The under lying bone may get exposed. Gangrene is denoted by blackening of the skin and presence of foul smell. The patients may develop toxemia.

Q80. What is Virus ?
Ans. Virus are submicroscopic particle containing nucleic acid and which reproduce only within specific living cells.

Q81. What are the types of Viruses ?
Ans. The viruses are classiffed as either RNA type of DNA depending on its structure. The viruses contain either Ribonucleic acid or Deoxyribonucleic acid. They are also subclassified depending on size, shape and structure.

Q82. What is the size of Viruses ?
Ans. The viruses are submicroscopic and may vary from 10 millimicron to 200 millimicrons.

Q83. Mention few RNA Viruses.
Ans. Paramyxovirus, Rhabdovirus, Picornavirus and Retrovirus are the few examples of RNA virus.

Q84. Mention few examples of DNA virus.
Ans. Herpes viruses, Poxviruses, Adenoviruses and Papovavirus are few examples of DNA virus.

Q85. Virus involved in AIDS belongs to which family of viruses ?
Ans. AIDS related virus belongs to DNA type (Cytomegalovirus).

Q86. What are the viruses grouped under herpesvires ?
Ans. Herpes simplex virus, Herpes zoster, cytomegalovirus, Epstein Barr virus are grouped under herpes group.

Q87. Which is the most commonest virus infection occurring in the body ?
Ans. Viral respiratory infection are the most commonest viral infections prevalent in human beings.

Q88. Which tissues are affected by herpes virus ?

Ans. Herpes virus commonly effects ectodermal derivatices like skin, mucous membrane, eyes and central nervous system.

Q89. What are the types of herpes simplex viruses ?
Ans. There are two immunologically different types of herpes simplex virus. They are type I affecting face, oral cavity and upper half of body and type II usually affecting lower half of the body including genitals.

Q90. What are the manifestations of herpes simplex infections ?
Ans. Herpes simplex viruses cause a severe form of disease which is known as primary herpetic gingivostomatitis and mild recurrent infection which is called recurrent or secondary herpes labialis.

Q91. Which age group is affected by primary herpetic gingivostomatitis ?
Ans. Children between 6 mnths and 6 years. Infants below 6 months are rarely affected as they are protected by maternal antibodies. Primary infection invariably cause immunity in old children.

Q92. Is it always essential to find positive history of acute herpetic stomatitis in individual exhibiting recurrent episodes of herpes labialis ?
Ans. No, Many individual suffer infection from herpes virus in childhood but without clinical symptoms. These are called subclinical infection. Such exposure to virus infection stinulate antibodies in the body and it is not necessary to find a positive history of acute primary infection.

Q93. What is herpetic whitlow ?
Ans. Herpetic whitlow is perpetic virus infection of finger or nails.

Q94. What are constitutional symptoms of primary herpes simplex infections ?
Ans. Primary attack invariably occurs in children, and is characterized by development of fever, irritability,

headache, pain while swallowing and regional lymphadenopathy. This is followed within few days by oral manifestations.

Q95. What are the major differences in clinical appearances in the ulcers of primary herpetic simplex and herpetic form aphthous ulcers ?

Ans. The herpetic form aphthous ulcers which occur on the nonkeratinized mucosa are multiple, circular and have a red halo whereas the ulcers in herpetic simplex are small and multiple in number and closed to each other. The aggression of ulcers cause appearance of long ulcerated area. The ulcers appear even in keratinized mucosa.

Q96. What are the oral manifestations of primary acute herpetic gingivostomatitis ?

Ans. Within few days of development of constitutional symptoms, the oral cavity becomes painful and gingival acutely inflamed. Oral Mucosa of tongue, cheeks, lips and pharynx may also be involved. Acute gingivitis is more prevalent. This is followed by appearance of tiny fluid filled vesicles. These vesicles rupture within hours leaving shallow painful ulcers. The ulcers vary in size however mostly they are small. These are surrounded by red halo. The ulcer are covered with grayish pseudombrane. The ulcers heals in 7 to 10 days without leaving any scars.

Q97. What is the type of vesicle in herpetic gingivostomatitis ?

Ans. The vesicles are superficial and are intraepithelial in location. They are filled with fluid in which many degenerating cells are found.

Q98. Describe the histologic picture of cells found in vesicles of acute herpetic gingivostomatitis.

Ans. The cells in vesicles exhibit either degeneration or other characteristic feature of intranuclear inclusion bodies. The degenerating cells show ballooning degeneration. The other cells exihibit eosinophilic, ovoid, homogeneous structure within the nucleus, which pushes nucleolus and nuclear chromatin to periphery. The intranuclear inclusion bodies are known as lipschutz bodies.

Q99. How do yhou manage a case of acute herpetic gingivostomatitis ?

Ans. The management of acute herpetic gingivostomatitis mostly is symptomatic and supportive. Treatment does not seem to alter the course of the disease but can reduce the symptoms. Therefore, use of alkaline mouth wash, and administration of analgesic and antipyretic drugs is advocated. Application of local antiseptic to prevent secondary infection. Bed rest and supportive therapy containing vitamin may be needed. Bland and liquid diet shall be given. Systemic use of antibiotics is advocated on few occasions to prevent secondary infection. Antiviral drugs like acyclovir can be given, however their use is limited for various reasons.

Q100. What is the reason for ineffectiveness of chemotherapy in herpetic gingivostomatitis ?

Ans. The herpes simplex virus does not remain latent at site. It reaches nerve ganglia supplying the area and remains latent over there. This incorporation of viral DNA into host cell DNA insures life long infection beyond the reach of antibodies or chemotherapy.

Q101. What are the precipitating factors for recurrent herpes infections ?

Ans. The latent herpes viruses become reactivated due to various factors. These include local trauma, exposure to sun rays, use of drugs, general debility, use of immunosuppressive drugs, fatigue, menstruation, hormonal changes, upper respiratory tract infection, gastrointestinal disturbances and emotional disturbances.

Q102. What are the clinical features of recurrent herpes simplex infection in oral cavity ?

Ans. The recurrent episode may occur very often or rarely with long intermission. The lesions may appear on lips or on mucosa within oral cavity. Most often it affects lips. Labial lesions are referred to as recurrent herpes labialis. On either locations, the appearance of vesicles is preceded by burning sensation, soreness, and inflammation at the site. The vesicles develop within next one or two days. Vesicles rupture leaving shallow ulcers. On lips these ruptured vesicles are covered by brownish crust.

Q103. Which locations of oral mucosa is mostly affected by recurrent herpes infection ?
Ans. Even though recurrent herpes virus affects lips most often, the intraoral lesions are not uncommon. Intraorally ulcers mostly occur on adherent mucosa or attached mucosa (keratinized mucosa). This is very important diagnostic differentiating point between the ulcers of recurrent herpeti ulcers of recurrent herpetic ulcers and recurrent aphthous ulcers. Recurrent aphthous ulcers usually occur on mobile or lining mucosa.

Q104. What are the other names of recurrent herpes labialis ?
Ans. Recurrent herpes labialis is also known as cold sores or cold blisters.

Q105. Mnetion few differences between ulcers of recurrent herpetic ulcers and recurrent aphthous ulcers.
Ans. Recurrent herpes ulcers occur on any part of oral mucosa including masticatory (Keratinised) mucosa whereas the aphthous ulcers occur on non keratinized epithelium and they appear more frequently. Recurrent herpetic lesions appears as vesicles and then rupture to form ulcer. Exposed surface of lips is the most commonest site for recurrent herpes ulceratior. It is usually followed by prodromal symptoms like fever, malaise before vesicles appear.

Q106. What is the difference between recurrent aphthous stomatitis and Aphthous pharyngitis ?
Ans. Recurrent aphthous stomatitis is common mucosal disorder with multiple etiological factors. It is simple and easy in

diagnosis but difficult to manage. The Aphthous pharyngitis is a specific viral disorder caused by Coxsackie group virus. It is also known as Herpangina and vesicular pharyngitis.

Q107. Write in brief the clinical features of herpangina.
Ans. Herpangina is a disorder of children. Affecrted children suffer from fever, vomiting, headache and muscular pains. These are associated with pharyngitis small vesicular eruption appear on pharyngeal and tonsillar mucosa. These vesicles break, leaving small ulcers covered by grayish slough and surrounded by red halo. They generally heal in about one week.

Q108. Which are the conditions one has to consider in differential diagnosis of small multiple ulcers of oral mucosa ?
Ans. In diagnosing the multiple small ulcers, one has to consider the following conditions in differential diagnosis. Herpangina, primary herpetic gingivostomatitis, Recurrent Aphthous ulcers, hand foot mouth disease, allergic stomatitis, cyclic neutropenia, and drythema multiform.

Q109. What are Koplik's spots ?
Ans. Koplik's spots are the intraoral manifestations seen in Measles. These are prodromal, and few in number and characterized by small bluish or whitish specks surrounded by red halo. These may appear on buccal mucosa and palate.

Q110. What are the other intraoral manifestations of measles ?
Ans. In addition to prodromal koplik's spots, the measles may cause pharyngitis, gingivitis and stomatitis. In addition to acute inflammation and congestion, ulcers may also appear.

Q111. What are the general manifestations of measles ?
Ans. The manifestations start to occur after incubation period of 8 to 10 days. Initially one may observe koplik's spots

intraorally. Measles is characterized by onset of fever, malaise, lacrimation, photophobia and cough. These are followed by paplar eruptions on skin. These begin on face and spreads downwards to extremities, neck chest and back. They coalesce to form patches. They disappear in 5 to 6 days.

Q112. What are the complications of Measles ?
Ans. Measles lowers the general body resistance leading to various systemic infections like pneumonia, encephalitis, otitis media and delay in healing of wounds etc. It may also cause immunosuppressive effect.

Q113. Which virus causes small pox ?
Ans. Small pox is an acute condition caused by variola.

Q114. How common is small pox now ?
Ans. Small pox is completely eradicated. It does not occur any more.

Q115. When was small pox completely eradicated ?
Ans. World Health Organization's global commission for the certification of eradication of small pox has made declaration of small pox eradication on ninth December 1979.

Q116. Which virus causes checken pox ?
Ans. Chicken pox is caused by varicella (Herpes zoster virus). It is an acute condition affecting children.

Q117. What is the incubation period for chcken pox ?
Ans. Incubation period for this acute and infectious disorder, chicken pox is about two weeks. Chicken pox is believed to be primary infection.

Q118. Write systemic clinical features of chicken pox.
Ans. Chicken pox commences with appearance of prodromal symptoms like headache, fever, pharyngitis, anorexia and malaise. The prodromal symptoms are followed by appearance oof maculopapular or vesicular eruptions of

the skin. They first occur on trunk and spread to face and extremities. The lesions rupture, forming superficial crusts and heal by desquamation. The disease may heal in 8 to 10 days.

Q119. Write oral manifestations of chicken pox and their differential diagnosis.
Ans. Oral lesions are uncommon. The oral mucosal lesions include appearance of vesicles on various parts including buccal, labial, palatal and pharyngeal mucosa nad gingival. The vesicles rupture leaving ulcers surrounded by inflammatory halo. These are multiple ulcers. Herpetic ulcers and recurrent Aphthous ulcers shall be considered in differential diagnosis.

Q120. What is shingles ?
Ans. Herpes zoster virus infection is also known as shingles. Herpes zoster is an acute and painful condition. It is believed that herpes zoster occurs due to reactivation of latent varicella virus which is acquired and remains dormant in the ganglian from previous infection.

Q121. Write the clinical features of herpes zosters.
Ans. Herpes virus disease is an acute inflammatory condition resulting in severe pain and vesicular or ulcerative lesions in the areas of skin and mucosa supplied by that particular nerve. It usually affects adults or elder persons. The onset of the disease is by appearance of prodromal symptoms like malaise, feer, and pain along the course of the nerve. The pain is limited to affected side (unilateral). Within few days of prodromal symptoms, papules or vesicles on skin or mucosa appear in linear arrangement along the course of the nerve. The vesicle may rupture resulting in ulcers. However in most of the cases, the herpes zoster virus is reactivated by certain precipitating factors. These are trauma, immunosuppression., malignancy, radiation, and stress. In orofacial region the herpes sozter may affect any of the three branches of trigeminal nerve. Vesicular eruptions along the distribution of affected branch occur.

Q122. How the differentiate the ulcers of herpes zoster from the ulcers of herpes simplex ?

Ans. Ulcers in herpes zoster characteristically always are located on one side and do not cross midline, whereas the ulcers of herpes simplex do not exihibit any characteristic distribution. Herpes zoster is associated with severe neuralagic pain in the course of nerve. Herpes zoster cannot be transmitted to animals (rabbits) whereas herpes simplex can be transmitted.

Q123. What are the clinical features of herpes zoster infection of geniculate ganglion ?

Ans. Reactivation of infection herpes zoster in geniculate ganglion results in facial muscles paralysis, appearance of vesicles on the external ear and sometimes on oral mucosa (oropharynx). Pain occurs in external and internal ear. These complex symptoms are referred as Ramsay Hunt syndrome.

Q124. Mention the various antiviral agents.

Ans. Antiviral agents are :
  For Herpes group : Idoxuridine, Vidarabine, Trifluridine, Acyclovir, Ganciclovir.
  For Retrovirus   : Zidovudine (AZT), Didanosine, Foscarnet.
  For Influenza A   : Amantadinie, Ribavirin.
  Non selective   : Human Interferons.
  Non selective   : Human Interferons.

Q125. Write the therapeutic doses of acyclovir.

Ans. 200 mg of Acyclovir given orally for every 4 hours (5 times a day) for 10 days.
  Ointment applied for every 3 hours, six times daily for 7 days.

Usual dose for treatment of infections of skin and mucous membrances in adults is 5 mg\kg every 8 hours for 7 days.

Q126. Write the prophylactic dose of acyclovir.
Ans. Long term suppressive therapy of recurrent disease in 30 mg, 3 to 5 times daily upto 6 months.

Q127. What is the complication of herpes zoster infection ?
Ans. Herpetic neuralgia characterized by severe burning and pain in areas supplied by nerve burning and pain in area supplied by nerve is the main complication of herpes zoster. Neuraligic attacks may occur repeatedly following precipitating factors like use of immunosuppressive angents, severe and chronic illness and lowered resistance. \

Q128. Which group of virus causes viral mumps ?
Ans. Paramyxovirus causes viral mumps.

Q129. What is the incubation period in viral mumps ?
Ans. Incubation period in viral mumps is two to three weeks.

Q130. Mention prodromal symptoms of viral mumps.
Ans. After incubation period of two to three weeks, the onset of viral mumps occurs with prodromal symptoms like fever, headache, vomiting ,malaise and pain in pre auricular region as commonest gland to be involved first is parotid gland.

Q131. Mention clinical features of viral mumps.
Ans. Viral mumps is an acute disorder affecting any major salivary glands. It may initially affect one gland and spread to others. Most often, the parotid gland is affected. The affected gland is enlarged and painful. Amount of saliva is reduced. Preauricular swelling with raised ear lobes is associated with parotid gland involvement. The ara appears tense. Patients complain of difficulty in mastication and swallowing and pain in gland. It is infectious disease, as virus is present in saliva.

Q132. What are the complications of viral mumps ?
Ans. The other organs may be affected as complications. The organs incude testis, pancreas and ovary. The orchitis may lead to sterility.

Q133. What are the management of viral Mumps.
Ans. Rest and symptomatic treatment like antipyretic and analgesics ar given. Sialogogues help in reduction in discomfort and prevention of retrograde infection. Antiviral drugs may be useful.

Q134. What are the other causes of Mumps ?
Ans. Viral mumps is specific disorder. There are other nonvirus causes for enlargement of salivary glands. These include bacterial, chronic nonspecific, nutritional and chemical mumps.

Q135. What is the bacterial parotitis ?
Ans. Parotitis or sialedenitis caused by bacteria is referred as bacterial parotitis. The infection may enter the glands through ductal opening, in patients suffering due to xerostomia caused by post surgical dehydration or chronically ill patients. Therefore, it is the also referred as postoperative parotitis, or surgical mumps or retrograde parotitis.

Q136. What is the etiology of chemical Mumps ?
Ans. Bilateral swelling of the salivary glands occasionally accompanies the administration of either or ganic or inorganic iodine. Therefore this is usually referred as "Iodine mumps" or Chemical mumps."

Q137. What is AIDS ?
Ans. AIDS is acronym for Acquired Immuno Deficiency Syndrome. It is symptom complex.

Q138. When was it first reported ?
Ans. AIDS cases were reported first in early eighties (1981). The reporting of first few cases was due to finding of severe infection due to pneumocystis carinii in previously otherwise healthy individuals. Earlier this infection was seen in mostly patients receiving immunosuppressive durgs for malignancies. Pneumocystis Carinii is opportunistic infection.

Q139. What is the etiology of AIDS ?
Ans. AIDS is caused by human immunodeficiency virus (HIV)

Q140. HIV belongs to which type of virus ?
Ans. HIV is a RNA retrovirus. It was formerly known as human T cell lymphotropic virus or lymphadenopathy associated virus.

Q141. Which group of individuals are more prone for AIDS ?
Ans. Transmission of AIDS most often found in homosexuals, bisexual males, intravenous drug abusers, Haemophilics and other individuals who receives blood often. These groups are "risk" groups. Heterosexual partners of such risk group also become prone for AIDS.

Q142. What are constitutional symptoms of AIDS ?
Ans. Constitutional symptoms in AIDS affected individuals are vague. These most often include unexplained generalized lymphadenopathy, swinging fever, weight loss, diarrhea, fatigue and joint pains. These are self limiting and may persist for few weeks only.

Q143. Which cells are more susceptible to HIV ?
Ans. T4 lymphocytes, monocytes and microglial cells are susceptible for HIV virus.

Q144. What is incubation period is AIDS ?
Ans. Constitutional symptoms appear 4 to 6 weeks after initial contact with HIV.

Q145. Describe the couse of AIDS.

Ans. Acute constitutional symptoms which persist for few weeks are self limiting and subside. The individuals remain asymptomatic for next 7 to 10 years. During this long duration or period the T4 lymphocytes deplete in number to such a low level that their count may reach 50 per cmm instead of 800 to 1200 per cmm in normal individuals.

Q146. What is the pathogenesis of generalized lymphadenopathy in AIDS ?

Ans. In individuals infected with HIV, there may be persistent generalized lymphadenopathy during asymptomatic phase. Unexplained, asymptomatic lymph node enlargement in more than 3 to 4 sites including cervical region seen in AIDS patients. The lymphadenopathy could be the result of nodal B lymphocytes attempting to contain virus.

Q147. What is ARC ?

Ans. ARC is acronym for AIDS related complex. The complex consist of occurrence of oral or vaginal condidiasis, hairy leukoplakia, herpes zoster or tuberculosis.

Q148. What are neurologic manifestations in AIDS ?

Ans. Neurologic manifestations in AIDS patients may occur anytime during the course of disease however they are severe in later period. These result from both direct infection of CNS with HIV or indirectly through opportunistic infections or neoplasms of brain. Common AIDS related CNS infections result from toxoplasmosis, Cryptococcus or cytomegalovirus. Among the meoplasms, B cell lymphoma is the major one. Direct infection of CNS by HIV will results in encephalopathy referred as AIDS dementia complex.

Q149. What is the significance of oral lesions in HIV infected patients ?

Ans. Even though the oral manifestations are specific lesions to HIV infections, these are very significant as they are often first sign of HIV infection. They have prognostic value.

Frequency and extensive involvement also should be kept in mind.

Q150. What are oral lesions in HIV infected patients ?
Ans. There are no primary lesions due to HIV infection. However there are many other opportunistic infections and lesions occur due to suppression of immunity. These are fungal, viral and bacterial infections, severe form of gingivitis and periodontitis and neoplasms.

Q151. Which fungal infections are related to HIV infections ?
Ans. Candidal infections, Cryptococcus and histoplasmosis are the fungal infections seen in AIDS patients. However candidiasis is most prevalent of the three. Pseudomembranous, atrophic, hyperplastic and angular cheilitis (Candidal) types of cnadidiasis occur in AIDS patients.

Q152. What is hairy leukoplakia ?
Ans. Hairy leukoplakia is white, corrugated or shaggy carpet like appearance, most often seen in lateral surface of toungue in AIDS patients. These are believed to be caused y opportunistic Epsteinbarr virus infection. The thick surface later peels of, leaving projections which resemble hair like projections.

Q153. Which viral infections are associated with HIV infected patients ?
Ans. Viral infections become opportunistic and effect in severe form in AIDS patients. Herpes simplex, herpes zoster, papillomavirus, Epstein barr virus and cytomegalovirus infections are the most often seen in AIDS patients.

Q154. What are the manifestations of cytomegalovirus ?
Ans. In AIDS patients, cytomegalovirus cause gastrointestinal disturbances, retinitis and oral ulcers. Histopathological examination of cells of these ulcerative lesions exhibit characteristic nuclear inclusion bodies.

Q155. Describe the gingival and periodontal diseases in AIDS patients.

Ans. Although most AIDS patients have periodontal disorders, which resemble the periodontal diseases seen in general population. Some AIDS patients exhibit severe characteristic gingival and periodontal diseases. The characteristic gingival and periodontal diseases. The characteristic gingivitis in AIDS patients presents as intense generalized erythematous gingivitis which does not respond to routine form of treatment. Acute necrotizing ulcerative gingivitis may be seen extensively.

HIV related periodontitis, spreads rapidly, causing intese destruction of periodontal tissues and alveolar bone causing loosening and loss of teeth.

Q156. What is Kaposi sarcoma ?

Ans. Kaposi sarcoma is a rare connective tissue neoplasm in elder population however it is most commonest of neoplasm found in AIDS patients. Kaposi sarcoma is also found in patients receiving immunosuppressive drugs for organ transplants. Kaposi sarcoma most frequently presents as vascular appearing macule, papule or nodule of mucosa or skin. Early lesions appear as ecchymosis or haemangioma. Disseminated form may involve gastrointestinal tract, lymph nodes or lungs.

Q157. Which other neoplasms may be seen in AIDS patients ?

Ans. Among the neoplasm, seen in AIDS patients Kaposi sarcoma is common than others. Other neoplasms include non Hodgkins lymphoma, Hodgkins lymphoma and cervical carcinoma.

Q158. Write histopathological appearance of Kaposi sarcoma.

Ans. Kaposi sarcoma presents a classical histological appearance. Well circumscribed mucocutaneous nodule composed of a dense mass of spindle shap3ed cells with thin vascular elements in between. Extravasation of erythrocytes and hemosiderin pigment deposition may be seen around thin wall3ed irregular blood vessels. Perivascular infiltration of lympyhocytes including plasma cells and numeruous eosinophilic bodies are diagnostic significant.

Q159. What is the risk incidence of health workers from AIDS patients ?
Ans. As HIV infection presented with multiple and various manifestation and proved fatal, fear of risk of contacting the disease while handling and managing these patients by various health workers was natural. This is compounded as HIV was found in saliva of AIDS patients. However it was found that infectivity of HIV to oral health workers was found to be very less compared to hepatitis B virus.

Q160. Which is the most commonest fungus which causes infection in orofacial region ?
Ans. Candida Albicans is the most commonest fungus which causes infection in oral cavity. Other species like candida tropicalis and candida parapsilosis may also infect.

Q161. Isolation of candida from smears of oral cavity indicate candidal infection. Is it true ?
Ans. No. The candida Albicans is common inhabitant of oral cavity, gastrointestinal tract and vagina. Mere Isolation of this organism does not indicate disease.

Q162. What is the criteria for detecting infection of candida ?
Ans. Penetration of deeper layers of mucosa by hyphae and increased concentration of candida shall be criteria for diagnosing candidiasis.

Q163. What is moniliasis ?
Ans. Moniliasis, or candidosis are the other names of candidiasis (Candidal infection).

Q164. What are the factors which cause candidal organisms to become pathogenic, even though they are common inhabitants in normal individuals ?

Ans. The candida albicans are found in the oral microbial flora. However candida is considered to be most opportunistic infection. The organisms become active in certain given favorable conditions. The favorable conditions are known as precipitating factors.

Q165. What are the various favorable or precipitating factors for candidiasis ?
Ans. The factors which precipitate candidiasis are (i) prolonged use of antibiotics which destroy and disturb normal microbial flora, (ii) prolonged illness, (iii) hormonal imbalance and disorders (diabetes etc.) (iv) use of immunosuppressive disorders (v) use of cytotoxic drugs in malignancies (vi) immune deficiency disorders, (vii) poor oral hygiene, (viii) poorly maintained dentures or orthodontic appliances, and (ix) radiation.

Q166. Is the candidias a keratotic or nonkeratotic white lesions ?
Ans. Candidal infection of oral mucosa may causeeither keratotic changes or nonkeratotic pseudomembrane. Both these conditions appear as white.

Q167. Classify the oral mucosal candidiasis.
Ans. Oral mucosal candidiasis can be classified as under
- I. Acute Candidiasis
    a. Acute pseudomemranous
    b. Acute Atrophic
- II. Chronic candidiasis
    a. Chronic hypplastic
    b. Chronic atrophic
    c. Chronic pseudomembranous
- III. Chronic mucocutaneous candidiasis.
    a. Chronic familial mucocutaneous candidiasis
    b. Chronic candidiasis endocrinopathy syndrome
    c. Chronic diffuse mucocutaneous candidiasis.

Q168. Describe acute pseudomembranous candidiasis.
Ans. Acute pseudomembranous candidiasis is also called thrush. It is a superficial acute infection caused by candida

albicans. It is scrapable as the white or yellowish patch can be easily removed. The white coating is made up of desquamated epithelial cells, inflammatory cells, fibrin, candida, and mycelia elements. Removal of pseudomembrane leaves raw, inflamed erosive areas of mucosa. Dorsal surface of tongue is most common site however the other areas may also be affected.

Q169. Which media is used to culture the candida ?
Ans. Candida albicans can be grown on Sabouraud's agar.

Q170. Which is the most often associated predisposing factor in acute atrophic candidiasis ?
Ans. Prolonged use of broad spectrum antibiotics is most often responsible predisposing factor which encourages multiplications of candida by suppressing other microbial growth. Acute atrophic candidiasis is also known as antibiotic sore mouth.

Q171. Write clinical features of acute atrophic candidiasis.
Ans. Acute atrophic candidiasis presents as erythematous patches which are painful with or without any evidence of pseudomembrane. Depapillation of tongue may be associated. Burning sensation, bad taste, and sore mouth are common features. These patients exhibit increased levels of antibody levels in serum.

Q172. Describe denture sore mouth.
Ans. Denture sore mouth is a diffuse inflammation of maxillary denture bearing oral mucosal surface. This is associated with poorly maintained dentures, and poorly fitting dentures. The mucosa appears inflamed, red, velvety and tender. The inflammation may show clear demarcation and localization to denture bearing area. The surface may bleed and painful. This may be associated with angular cheilitis. Antibody titres in serum and saliva are faised. Three varieties of denture sore mouth are described. They are (a) localised simple or pinpoint inflammatory areas (b) more diffused area of inflammation and (c) granular or papillary eruptions associated with inflamed mucosa.

Q173. Describe chronic hyperplastic candidiasis.
Ans. Chronic hyperplastic candidiasis is also sometimes referred as candidial leukoplakia is a chronic condition exhibiting deeper invasion of mycelia of fungus and cellular chages in epithelium. The epithelium may show hyperkeratosis or parakeratosis, acanthosis, mocroabscess formation and infiltration of chronic inflammatory cells. The hyphae can be demonstrated by staining with P.A.S.

Clinically it presents as firm, leathery, white plaque or patch on buccal, labial or lingual mucosa. It is non scrapable white lesion. Candidial leukoplakia is at higher risk for changes occurring as carcinoma as it is observed that dysplastic changes in epithelium occur four or five times more frequently than in leukoplakia.

Q174. What is Id reaction ?
Ans. Some patients with chronic cnadiasis develop a secondary skin response characterized by a localised or generalized sterile vesiculopapular eruptions. These lesions which are referred to as monilids or Id reaction, generally resolve after the treatment of candidiasis. This is believed to be an allergic reaction to candida antigens.

Q175. What is candida hypersensitivity syndrome ?
Ans. Candida hypersensitivity syndrome consists of an ill defined group of symptoms, like fatigue, gas trointestinal disturbances, headache, premenstrual symptoms, and rashes. These are believed to be due to candidal infection of oral, gastrostinal of vaginal mucosa.

Q176. Mention various antifungal agents.
Ans. The various agents have been sued as antifungal agents. These include dye like gentian violet. Mouth wash like chlorhexidine mouth wash, imidazole derivatives like clotrimazole, miconazole, ketoconazole and fluconazole, antibiotics like nystatin and amphotericin B.

Q177. Mention the antifungal drugs which can be given intravenously ?

Ans. Fluconazole and amphotericin B can be sued in travenously.

Q178. Mention the antifungal drugs used as topical applications.
Ans. Nystatin (Oral suspension and cream), clotrimazole (troches and cream), gentian violet, and chlorhexidine are used as topical agents.

Q179. Mention the uses of nystatin.
Ans. Nystatin is used in the treatment of candida infections. It is used either as cream or as an oral suspension or sucrose containing oral pastille for slow release, or lactose containing vaginal tablets allowed to dissolve slowly under the tongue.
Nystatin is available as oral suspension in the dose of 100000 units per ml nystatin pastilles (200000 units per pastille) and nystatin cream 1%.

Q180. What are the side affects of using nystatin tablets or pastilles ?
Ans. Nystatin tablets contain lactose and nystatin pastille contain sucrose. These are allowed to remain in oral cavity for slow releae of drug for local effect. Hence the sucrose and lactose are potential cariogenic agents.

Q181. What is the dose of ketoconazole ?
Ans. Ketoconazole is used as 200 mg tablet once or twice a day, for one to two weeks.

Q182. What is the dose of fluconazole ?
Ans. Fluconazole is prescribed as 100 mg tablet once or twice a day.

Q183. What are the side effects of fluconazole ?
Ans. Long use of fluconazole may produce pain and pruritis.

Q184. What are the aspects considered in management of oral candidiasis ?
Ans. In the management of oral candidiasis, selection of antifungl medication, its mode of use and dosage are

important. In addition to use of antifungal agents. Attention also shall be given to prevent or correct predisposing and precipitating factors which encourage candidal infection.

Q185. How do you manage a case of chronic atrophic candidiasis associated with wearing of dentures ?
Ans. Chronic atrophic candidiasis associated with dentures (denture sore mouth) is a conditions seen in older persons and is associated with ill fitting and poorly maintained dentures. Topical applicaton of nystatin cream on mucosa and suspension of denture in antifungal solution for few days may help. Denture can be worn after applying the cream. In severe form many require relining of the denture. Therefore treatment shall be directed to both the affected tissues as well as dentures.

Q186. Which factor enhances rapid and better absorption of ketoconazole from stomach ?
Ans. Presence of acid in stomach enhances the absorption of ketoconazole. In patients suffering from achlorhydria, acidified solution of ketoconazole shall be used.

Q187. Which drugs interfere with absorption of ketoconazole ?
Ans. Antacids, anticholinergic agents and histamine H2 blockers are the some drugs which interfere with absorption of ketoconazole. Hence ketoconazole shall be administered after a gap of 2 3 hours.

Q188. What are the durgs which may interact with fluconazole and limit their use ?
Ans. Fluconazole interacts with number of drugs including anticoagulants, phenytoin, cyclosporine, antihistamines and oral hypoglycemic drugs. Therefore proper care shall be taken while using fluconazole and other drugs.

Q189. What is Darling's disease ?
Ans. Darling's disease is histoplasmosis. It is a fungal disease caused by organism histoplasma capsulatum.

Q190. Write clinical features of histoplasmosis.
Ans. Histoplasmosis may occur as generalized form or as a local form in few occasion. Generalised form is charcterised by low grade fever, productive cough, splenomegaly, hepatomegaly, and lymphadenopathy. As the organism has special affinity to reticuloendothelial system, lymph nodes, spleen, liver and bone marrow are involved. As a results of involvement of bone marrow, anemia and leucopenia also may be present. The local lesions may cause subcutaneous nodules or suppurative arthritis.

Q191. Give the oral manifestations of histoplasmosis.
Ans. The lesions may occur on buccal mucosa, gingival, tongue and palate. The lesions may appear as nodular, ulcerative or vegetating. The ulcerative lesions are usually covered by gray pseudomembrane. Microorganisms may be isolated from the lesions.

Q192. What is the incidence of cryptococcosis ?
Ans. Even though the organisms (fungus) cryptococus neoformans and Cryptococcus bacillospora are found to be frequently present on the skin of healthy individuals, the infection is not very conmmon. However the incidence is more where immunosuppression has occurred.

Q193. Give the clinical feature of cryptococcosis infection.
Ans. First evidence of infection is usually includes papules on the skin which may ulcerate and the infection disseminates from skin to other parts through blood stream. Infection lung may present as nonspecific pneumonitis. While meningeal involvement causes variety of neurological signs.
Cryptococcosis is an opportunistic infection. Hence found to occur in patients suffering from malignant lymphoma, and immunosuppression.

Q194. Mention the manifestations of cryptococcosis.

Ans. Oral manifestations are uncommon. However the oral lesions are seen in patients having systemic manifestations.

The oral lesions are nonspecific and appear as single or multiple ulcers on tongue, buccal mucosa and lips.

Q194. Write the morphological characteristics of cryptococcosis.

Ans. The fungus Cryptococcus, is gram positive, budding, yeast like cell. It has thick gelatinous capsule. The Cryptococcus measures 5 to 20 microns. The capsule is intensely stained with P. A. S.

Q196. Write the microscopic appearance of Cryptococcus lesions.

Ans. The tissue reaction to cryptococcus infection is usually a granulomatous one of tuberculous type but focal necrosis is absent and epitheloid cell proliferation is minimal. Multinucleated giant cells are common. The organism in tissue may be seen as dense small organism with a large clear halo. These cells may be present either singly or in groups, scattered throughout the granuloma.

5.

DENTAL CARIES

Q1. Define dental caries.
Ans. Dental caries is a microbial disease of calcified tissue of teeth, characterized by demineralization of the inorganic portion and destruction of organic part of hard tissues.

Q2. Which sex is more prone for caries ?
Ans. Incidence of caries is observed in both the sexes equally.

Q3. Which age group is more prone for caries ?
Ans. Children and young adults exhibit more incidence of dental caries.

Q4. Which teeth show high incidence of caries ?
Ans. Dental caries affects most often mandibular first molars and followed by maxillary first molars. Second molars come next in incidence of caries.

Q5. Which teeth have lower incidence of dental caries ?
Ans. Canines are least affected by dental caries.

Q6. What could be the reason for higher incidence of caries in molars ?
Ans. The reasons for higher incidence of caries in molars could be their posterior locations, their morphology of having more pits and fissures and early eruption of first molars in oral cavity.

Q7. Which surface of molar teeth shows higher incidence of caries?

Ans. Occlusal surface is more prone for development of caries, followed by mesial, distal, buccal and lingual surfaces in diescending order.

Q8. Classify dental caries.
Ans. DENTAL caries is classified in a number of ways, like based on location, rapidity of progress, based on occurrence and based of tissues involved.

Q9. Classify dental caries based on location.
Ans. Based on location of carries, the dental caries can be classified either as pit and fissure caries or as smooth surface caries.

Q10. Classify the dental caries based on rapidity of progress.
Ans. Based on rate of progress, the caries is classified as acute caries, chronic caries and arrested caries. Rampant carries including nursing bottle caries is a acute form of dental caries.

Q11. Classify the caries based on occurrence.
Ans. Based on occurrence, the dental caries is classified ether as primary (on intact surface) or as secondary or recurrent (around restorations).

Q12. Classify the caries based on tissues involved.
Ans. The caries is classified based on tissues involved as enamel caries, dentinal caries and cemental caries (root caries).

Q13. Write in brief the clinical features of caries.
Ans. Dental caries may present in different forms depending on the extension of involvement. The appearance may vary from mild chalky white appearance to large brownish or dark cavity. The appearance differs from smooth surface to pit and fissure.

Q14. Give the clinical features of primary caries of smooth surface.

Ans. Primary caries of smooth surface occurs mostly on proximal surface of teeth, cervical thirds of buccal and lingual surfaces of posteriors and labial surface of incisors. The development of caries on these surfaces is preceded by formation of dental plaque. Proximal caries usually begins just below the contact point and appears in the early stages as a faint white opacity of the enamel surface. In some areas it appears as a yellow or brown pigmented areas. These early lesions become slightly roughened owning to decalcification of enamel. Extension of caries below the proximal enamel ridge, gives rise to bluish appearance. Later as extension occurs cavity formation is common with loss of contact point patients complain of food stagnation, hypersensitivity, and later paibn on mastication due to pressure of impacted food on interdental gingival. Deeper penetration of caries to dentin may lead to pulpal diseases.

Q15. Describe the clinical features of primary caries of pit and fissure.

Ans. Primary caries of pit and fissure develops on occlusal surfaces of premolars and molars, buccal surfaces of molars and lingual surfaces of maxillary incisors. Deep, narrow pits and fissures favour retention of the food debris and microorganisms, which on fermentation result in acid and demineralization.

These areas of initial caries appear brown or balck and will feel soft and yielding to probing. Caries may spread laterally below enamel. Enamel over such undermining carious lesion appear bluish. The caries may spread laterally along with the dentinoenamel junction and deeper into dentine along with dentinal tubules. Thus a large carious lesion may be found below with very tiny opening at surface of overlying enamel. The unsupported enamel may break due to masticatory forces or due to manipulation by dental surgeon, exhibiting a large cavity.

Q16. What are the clinical features of cervical caries ?

Ans. Cervical caries mostly occurs in gingival third of buccal, lingual, and labial surfaces. It spreads laterally. Typical cavity is described as crescent shaped cavity near the gingival margin. The incidence of cervical caries is very uncommon as the areas is self cleansing area and food dies not get stagnated easily.

Q17. What is acute dental caries ?
Ans. Acute dental caries is that form of caries which runs a rapid clinical course and results in early pulp involvement by carious process.

Q18. What is rampant caries ?
Ans. Rampant caries, is an acute form of caries, which affects multiple teeth and spreads rapidly.

Q19. What is nursing bottle caries ?
Ans. Nursing bottle caries, also called baby bottle syndrome and bottle mouth syndrome is a form of rampant caries affecting deciduous teeth. The cause has been attributed to prolonged use of feeding bottle containing milk, milk products or sweetened fruit juices, or sweetened water. This is often used as an aid to induce sleep and bottle is allowed to remain for longer duration. Deciduous maxillary incisors, molars and canines are affected by caries. The mandibular incisors are free from caries. This is probably due to protection given by protruding tongue which covers the mandibular teeth.

Q20. Give examples of rampant caries.
Ans. Nursing bottle caries and caries seen in patients with history of radiation exposure to facial region, are the good examples of rampant caries. Rapidly occurring caries involving multiple teeth is seen in patients suffering with xerostomia due to radiation exposure of salivary glands. This is also referred to as radiation caries.

Q21. What is chronic caries ?
Ans. Chronic dental caries is that form which proresses slowly and is most often seen in adults. The entrance to the

lesion is larger than seen in acute caries. Probably due to wider opening, food does not get retained and saliva also can reach the area easily. The slow progress is due probably to narrow dentinal tubules, formation of reparative dentine and deposition of secondary dentine. The lesion is usually dark brown.

Q22. Describe the recurrent caries.
Ans. Recurrent caries is the caries which occurs around restorations. It could be due to inadequate removal of originally involved tooth substance, inadequate condensation of restoration leaving gaps, poor adaptation of filling material to cavity causing marginal leakage.

Q23. What is arrested caries ?
Ans. Arrested caries is name given to carious lesion, which becomes static and which do not show any further progress.

Q24. Describe arrested caries.
Ans. Arrested caries is carious lesion which remains static and does not show any tendency for progress. It is relatively uncommon. It can be seen both in deciduous and permanent dentition. It can be seen on occlusal surfaces and is characterized by a large open cavity in which there is lack of food retention and in which superficially softened and decalcified dentin is gradually burnished until it takes brownish, polished, smooth shallow appearance. The surface is hard.
Arrested caries can also on proximal surfaces of teeth in which adjacent approximating tooth is removed. The caries does not spread as food stagnation is no more present. The arrested caries appears as an yellow or brown stained area below the contact point.

Q25. What is "consolidation of caries ?
Ans. Consolidation of caries is also referred to as reversibility of caries. It is process of remineralisation of early carious lesions due to local application of stannous fluoride solutions. The remineralisation processor from the minerals

from saliva, or as a result of fluoride ions stimulating increased deposition of calcium phosphate on tooth surface.

Q26. What is the etiology of dental caries ?
Ans. The dental caries results from complex problems associated as direct and indirect factors. There are variety of factors which play significant role in causing caries. The process and role of these factors are described in the form of theories of dental caries.

Q27. What are the theories of dental caries ?
Ans. There are three theories dental caries. They are (a) Acidogenic theory (b) proteolytic theory and (c) proteolysis-chelation theory.

Q28. Describe acidogenic theory.
Ans. Acidogenic theory or Miller's chemico-parasitic theory proposes that dental caries is a chemicoparasitic process consisting of two stages, the decalcification of enamel and dentine and followed by dissolution or destruction of organic residue. The acid which affects the decalcification is produced from the fermentation of the starches and sugars by the microorganisms.

Q29. Which microorganisms cause fermentation of starch and sugars in causation of dental caries ?
Ans. Variety of microorganism are considered to be associated with fermentation of food. These include main group of lactobacillus acidophilus and Streptococcus mutans and Bacillus necrodental is.

Q30. Which carbohydrates are cariogenic ?
Ans. Carbohydrates which are readily fermentable by microorganisms are cariogenic. Sucrose, sugar and cooked starches produce more acids when fermented. The cariogenicity of dietary carbohydrate varies with the frequency of ingestion, physical form, chemical composition, route of administration and presence of other food constituents. Carbohydrate in the form of sticky solid

food, and soft sticky food are more acidogenic than in liquid form. Polysaccharides are less easily fermented than monosaccharides and disaccharides.

Q31. Which acid is responsible for development of dental caries ?
Ans. The fermentation of carbohydrate by microorganisms will produce acid. Mostly these are lactic acid and butyric acid.

Q32. What is dental plaque ?
Ans. Dental plaque is a thin pellicle of deposition on tooth surface. It consists of salivary component, mucin, desquamated epithelial cells, and microorganisms.

Q33. What is microcosm ?
Ans. Dental plaque is also called microcosm.

Q34. What is sordes ?
Ans. Sordes is whitish gummy material discharged from gingival crevices and generally observed in fever and patients with poor oral hygiene.

Q35. What is critical pH of dental plaque for initiation of decalcification ?
Ans. Decalification of enamel under dental plaque commences when pH falls between 4.0 to 5.5 pH.

Q36. What is proteolytic theory of dental caries ?
Ans. This thory postulates that it is organic component which is affected first by proteolytic enzymes. It is believed that microbial gain entry through enamel lamellae and cause destruction by proteolytic enzymes or acids.

Q37. Describe proteolysis-chelation theory.
Ans. The proteolysis-chelation theory of dental caries is proposed by Schatz and his associates. It states that the caties is initiated by keratinolytic microorganisms causing break down of organic component of enamel mostly keratin. This results in production of substances which may form soluble chelates with the mineralized component of

the tooth and thereby decalcify the enamel even at neutral or alkaline pH.

Q38. What are the tooth related factors which influence dental caries ?

Ans. Composition, morphologic characteristics, and position of teeth are the factors which influence the occurrence and progress of dental caries.

Q39. How does the composition of tooth affect the dental caries ?

Ans. Number of studies on relation of etiology of caries to chemical composition of teeth were conducted. No significant differences were found in calcium, phosphorus, magnesium and carbonate contents of enamel from sound and carious teeth. However fluoride content was found to be significantly low in carious teeth. It is also significant finding that surface of enamel is highly mineralized with chemicals like fluoride, zinc, lead, and iron. Therefore surface is more resistant to development of caries. Further surface of enamel is lower in carbondioxide and dissolves at a slower rate in acids.

Q40. How do the morphological characteristics of teeth influence the occurrence of caries ?

Ans. Hypoplastic teeth are more prone to caries development. Teeth with deep pits and fissures which help in food stagnation, also more prone for development of caries. Deep lingual pits on maxillary incisors also mae them more prone for development of caries.

Q41. How does the tooth position influence the occurrence of caries ?

Ans. Tooth position in the arch plays a vital role in caries occurrence. Malpositioning, crowding, impaction makes the teeth more prone for caries as the food stagnation and food retention occurs in the narrow spaces. Caries can develop in such areas of food retention.

Q42. Describe the role of saliva in causation of dental caries.

Ans. The teeth are in constant contact with the saliva. This local environment of presence of saliva, may influence the occurrence of various deseases including caries. Numerous studies were conducted on the role of various constituents of saliva to the incidence of caries. The concentration of calcium, phosphorus, was found to be low in individuals with high caries rate. Ammonia content was found to be high in caries free individuals. However these findings were not confirmed in other studies.

The quantity of saliva may have significant role in caries activity. In individuals suffering with xerostomia, incidence of caries was found to be more and spread of caries is rapid. Caris prone individual exhibited more viscous saliva.

The buffer capacity of the saliva received considerable attention of investigators for its role in incidence of caries. It is observed that variation in pH of saliva did not show much significance. However the lo pH under dental plaque and at the site of caries was a significant finding.

Q43. How does enamel caries of smooth surface differs from enamel caries of pit and fissure ?

Ans. Enamel caries of smooth surface differs from the enamel of pit nd fissure in its spread and shape of cavity. In smooth surface caries, the decay starts at wider area and spreads along with enamel rods dentino-enamel junction in a triangular form. The wider base being towards surface of enamel and apex being towards dentino-enamel function. In the caries of pit and fissure, the lesion commences as a tiny, subclinical perforation of enamel surface at the base of pit and spreads towards dentinoenamel junction in a triangular shape as well. However triangular cavity is arranged in reverse order. The apex is towards surface enamel and wider base is towards dentino-enamel junction.

Q44. Describe the microscopic appearance of enamel caries of smooth surface.

Ans. Microscopically, the different zones can be distinguished in enamel caries the zone from dentinal side are as follows.

Zone-1: Advancing zone of caries of enamel near the dentine is seen and enamel in this zone is more porous than sound enamel. The pore volume being 1% whereas it is 0.1% in sound enamel.

Zone-2: Dark zone lies above the translucent one. The dark zone is formed due to demineralization of enamel.

Zone-3: This zone represents the bulk of body of carious lesion. It shows pore volume may range between 5% to 25%.

Zone-4: This is surface zone, appears relatively unaffected as the surface layer exhibits greater mineralization and greater concentration of fluoride.

Q45. Write microscopic changes of early caries of dentine.

Ans. Spread of caries from enamel to underlying dentine may occur faster in pit and fissure caries than smooth surface caries. The early changes include fatty degeneration of odontoblastic processes. The fatty goblets in dentinal tubules can be demonstrated by application of special stain like Sudan red. The initial decalcification involves the walls of the tubules, allowing them to distend slightly as they become packed with masses of microorganisms. Th4e widening of dentinal tubules is described as headed appearance. Tiny "Liquefaction foci" described by miller, are formed by focal coalescence and breakdown of dentinal tubules. Disintegated and softened dentine gives appearance of tiny areas which are described as transverse clerfts.

Q46. Describe the various zones seen in caries of dentine.

Ans. The changes occurring in dentine during the progress of carious lesion are seen as different zones. These are described pulpal side to enamel side.

Zone-1: Zone of fatty dgeneration of Tome's processes.

Zone-2: Zone of Sclerosis of dentine due to deposition of calcium salts in dentinal tubules. This reaction is defense mechanism and is an attempt to stop further progress of carious process. This zone is prominent in slowly progressing caries and may be absent in very rapidly progressing caries.
Zone-3: Zone of decalcification of dentin.
Zone-4: Zone of microbial invasion in decalcified but still intact dentine.
Zone-5: Zone of disintegrated and decomposed dentine.

Q47. How does the carious process of secondary dentine differe from primary dentine ?
Ans. Caries of secondary dentine basically does not differ from primary dentine, except that it is slow as the number of dentinal tubules is considerably less in secondary dentine.

Q48. Describe the rot caries.
Ans. Root caries is also referred as caries of cementum. Root caries occurs if the root surface is exposed to exterior due to gingival recession in older people or due to periodontal diseases. Formation of dental plaque and microbial invasion is essential. However it is observed that microorganisms involved are different from that of coronal caries, being filamentous rather than coccal.

The microorganisms invade the fibers or between these bundles of fibers. The microorganism try to spread laterally between the layers of cementum and caries of cementum results in decalcification and then destruction of cementum.

Q49. What is sclerotic dentine ?
Ans. Deposition of calcium salts in dentinal tubules occurs in dentin, pulpally to carious lesion of dentine or severe abrasion, attrition or erosion involving the dentine. Calcium deposition invariably preceded by fatty degeneration of Tome's processes in dentinal tubules. Thus the mineralization of tubules results in uniform refactive index, and dentine appears transparent or sclerotic in ground section. Tubules are not evident in sclerotic dentin.

Sclerotic dentine results not only from injury to the dentine by caries, abrasion, or attrition but also as a manifestation of normal ageing process.

Q50. What is reparative dentine ?

Ans. Reparative dentine is the dentine which is formed in response to severe form of irritation from any source. This is also called tertiary dentine, adventitious, and irritation dentine. It differs form secondary dentine as it contains lesser and irregular tubules and found at the pulpal end at the site of irritation.

6.

DISEASE OF PULP AND PERIAPICAL TISSUE

Q1. What are the etiological factors in pulp diseases?
Ans. Etiological factors in diseases of pulp include microbial invasion, trauma to the tooth, thermal injury, chemical injury, and electrical injury. The bacterial invasion may occur as result of microbial migrating from carious lesions or microbial invading the pulp directly in exposed pulp due to injuries or microbial may invade pulp through hematogenous route. Hematogenous infection is referred as "Anachorexia".

Q2. What is "Aerodontalgia"?
Ans. It is relatively uncommon condition. Aerodontalgia is a condition simulating pulpitis by occurrence of pain in tooth while flying in high attitudes. The pain is felt mostly in recently filled tooth or teeth.

Q3. How does the restorative procedures cause injury to the pulp?
Ans. Injury to pulp during restorative procedures may be caused either by cutting procedures or by the various filling materials used.

Q4. How do the use of burs to prepare the crown / cavity cause pulp injury?
Ans. Heat is generated by revolving, cutting and grinding instruments used in operative procedures. Heat causes injury to the pulp. The thermal changes may be influenced by the size, shape and composition of bur or stone, speed, amount and direction of pressure applied while cutting, the length of time the bur is in contact with the tooth, the

amount of moisture in the field of operation and the type of tissue being cut (enamel or dentine).

Q5. Other than cutting procedures, what are the other sources of heat, which may cause injury to pulp ?

Ans. In addition to heat generated during use of burs or stones for cutting the cavity or crown, the heat may also be generated during setting of various filling materials, particularly direct resins.

Q6. What are the preventive measures one can take to reduce heat generation during cavity preparation ?

Ans. There are various measures which can reduce the heat generation. These are use of water spray while cutting, use of high speed instruments. Use of small size burs or stones and decreased pressure on cutting surface are the various measures which can reduce heat generation.

Q7. What is rebound response observed in pulp while preparing a cavity?

Ans. Use of high instrument for cavity preparation cause changes like alteration in ground substance, edema, fibrosis, odontoblastic disruption, and reduced predentine formation in the pulp in the region directly across the cavity or at a distant site. This is believed to be caused b waves of energy transmitted to pulp focused into a certain region by pulpal walls. This is called rebound response of pulp.

Q8. What is calciotraumatic phenomena ?

Ans. A hyperchromatic line may develop along the pulpal margin of the dentin, concomitant with changes in the odontoblastic layer. This is known as calciotraumatic response.

Q9. How do the zinc oxyphosphate and silicate cement restorations affect the pulp ?

Ans. These cements cause hperaemia of pulp, destruction of odontoblasts, inflammation of pulp, and some times pulp abscess. The offending agent is phosphoric acid. Silicate cement is more injurious, than zinc oyphosphate cement because the mixing technique allows more free acid in silicate cement.

Q10. How does the self polymerizing acrylic resincause pulp damage ?
Ans. Monomer of the self polymerizing acrylic resin is offending agent for pulp damage.

Q11. Classify pulp disease.
Ans. The pulp diseases are classified in many ways, based either on nature of reaction (acute or chronic), or on extent of involvement (partial or total) or on extent of involvement (partial or total) or on presence or absence of communication (open or close). The following is the classification of pulp diseases.
I. Inflammatory
    (i)   Hyperaemia (Reversible Focal pulpitis)
    (ii)   Pulitis
    (A) Acute (a) Open (b) closed
    (B) Chronic (a) open type including chronic hyperplastic pulpitis (b) closed type.
II. Degenerative
    (i)   Reticular degeneration
    (ii)   Fibrous degeneration
    (iii) Calcifications (True, false and diffused)
    (iv) Necrosis
    (v)   Gangrene.

Q12. What is Focal reversible pulpitis ?
Ans. It is an earliest stage or form of pulpitis. The mild inflammatory changes are reversible and pulp reverses to normal appearance. The Focal reversible pulpitis or pulp hyperaemia can result from irritation to dentine and pulp or result from mild trauma. It is more often localized near the irritated dentinal tubules.

Q13. Write clinical features of Focal reversible pulpitis.
Ans. A tooth with Focal reversible pulpitis becomes sensitive to thermal stimuli. The pain disappears once the irritant is

withdrawn and normal temperatre is restored. The tooth responds to electrical pulp testing at lower level.

Q14. Describe the microscopic changes occurring in pulp hyperaemia.

Ans. Focal reversible pulpitis pulpal hyperaemia is characterized by dilatation of the blood vessels, extravasation red blood cells, and diapedesis of white blood cells. Transudation of fluid from blood vessels may occur leading to hemoconcentration of blood in vessels.

Q15. What is open acute pulpitis ?

Ans. Extensive, severe inflammation of pulp which has communication to exterior either through large carious lesions, or loss of enamel and dentitine due to mechanical injuries, attritrion, abrasion and erosion.

Q16. What is closed acute pulpitis ?

Ans. Severe form of inflammation in pulp of a tooth with intact dentinal wall is referred as closed acute pulpitis. Signs and symptoms are more severe and intense in closed type than in open type.

Q17. Write clinical features of acute pulpitis.

Ans. In acute pulpitis, invariably the onset is sudden. The tooth becomes very sensitive to thermal changes. The pain remains even after removal of stimulation. The pain is continuous, severe, aggravated by thermal changes, radiating type, and may be felt on whole half of the face. The patient usually fails to locate the offending tooth. Electrical pulp testing elicits response at lower current. The pain is more severe and lancinating when the entrance to the pulp is not wide open and pressure within the pulp tissue builds up due to accumulation of inflammatory fluid. The tooth with acute pulpitis is not sensitive to percussion unless inflammatory exudates escapes to apical region through apical foramen.

Q18. Describe microscopic changes in acute pulpitis.
Ans. Acute pulpitis is characterized by accumulation of edema, dilatation of blood vessels, pavementing of polymorphonuclear leukocytes, and their migration through the endothelial walls, into the surrounding connective tissues. Odontoblasts at the offending tubules get destroyed and pulpal tissue is infiltrated with white blood cells. Pus may result with destruction of microbial, leuk-cytes and pulpal tissue. The collection of pus may result in pulp abscess. Under microscope, the abscess may appear as empty space surrounded by pulp with numerous leukocytic infiltration.

Q19. Describe the clinical feature of chronic pulpitis.
Ans. Chronic pulpitis may result either through quiescence of a previous acute pulpitis or as chronic form its onset itself. The signs and symptoms are considerably milder than in acute form. Pain is not a prominent feature however many a times patients do complain of mild, dull and continuous pain in offending tooth. Tooth is not tender. Response to thermal changes considerably reduced and variant from time to time. Electrical pulp tester elicits delayed response.

Q20. What is chronic hyperplastic pulpitis ?
Ans. Chronic hyperplastic pulpitis or pulp polyp is a form of open type of chronic pulpitis in which there is excessive proliferation of inflamed pulp tissue.

Q21. What are the clinical features of chronic hyperplastic pulpitis ?
Ans. This condition is also called pulp polyp. It occurs almost exclusively in children and young adults and seen in teeth with large and open carious cavities. The teeth most commonly involved are deciduous molars and first permanent molars. Hperplastic pulp appears as pinkish red protruding tissue from caries cavity. The pulpal tissue fills up the cavity. The protruding pulp tissue is painless and insensitive to manipulation. It most often occurs in large occlusal surface cavities but may also occur in proximal caries cavities shall be differentiated from localized

papillary gingival growth which may occupy the proximal caries cavity.

Q22. Write the microscopic picture of pulp polyp.
Ans. Pulp polyp is a hyperplastic tissue basically granulation tissue made up of delicate connective tissue fibers, numerous small capillaries, and inflammatory cell infiltration. Fibroblast and endothelial cell proliferation may be seen in some areas. The granulation tissue becomes epithelised by the desquamated epithelial cells of oral mucosa, which become grafted on pulp polyp.

Q23. What are the sequelae of chronic pulpitis ?
Ans. Exacerbation of chronic pulpitis may result in acute phase. However the chronic pulpitis may result in necrosis of pulp, apical periodontitis, apical abscess, alveolar abscess and osteomyelitis. All these conditions need not follow in that order.

Q24. What are the sequelae of Necrosis of pulp ?
Ans. Sequelae of necrosis of pulp include apical periodontitis, apical abscess, alveolar abscess, osteomylitis, periapical granuloma and periapical cyst.

Q25. What is gangrene of pulp ?
Ans. Necrosis of pulp associated with bacterial infection is called gangrene. It can be dry or wet gangrene.

Q26. How does dry gangrene of pulp occurs ?
Ans. Gangrene of pulp occurring slowly and allowing the fluid to escape results in dry angrene. It is nonpurulent.

Q27. How does we gangrene occurs ?
Ans. Wet gangrene results from sudden occlusion of apical vessels. The pulp undergoes necrosis in presence of bacteria. Exudation does not drain away.
Necrosis, and gangrene of pulp are asymptomatic, however tooth in which pulp is undergoing gangrene may exhibit certain symptoms due to production of gases.

Q28. What is reticular atrophy of pulp ?
Ans. Regressive change or degenerative change occurring in aged pulp is described as reticular atrophy. The teeth are clinically asymptomatic. Reticular atrophy is characterized by the presence of large vacuolated spaces in the pulp, degeneration of odontoblast and reduction of cellular elements.

Q29. What is the incidence of pulp calcification ?
Ans. Various forms of claficiation are not ncommon in pulpal tissue. Almost 60% teeth exhibit pulp calcification in younger individuals ranging from 20 to 30 years. Whereas the incidence of pulp calcification in older persons may be around 80 to 90%. Teeth with small calcificatons usually are asymptomatic.

Q30. Classify pulp calcification ?
Ans. The pulp calcifications can be classified into (a) True (b) false and (c) diffuse calcification. The true and false pulp stones are again subdivided into either as free or attached or embedded depending on the location.

Q31. Describe true denticles.
Ans. True denticles are calcified masses in pulp which structurally resemble dentine. These exhibit tubular structure. True pulp stones have greater resemblance to secondary dentine than primary dentine as number of tubules are less in number and irregularly arranged. These stones are not common finding. They may occur near apical foramen. It is believed that cell rests of Malassez get entrapped into radicular pulp during formation of root. These cells give rise to true pulp stones.

Q32. Classify true pulp stones based on location ?
Ans. True pulp stones which structurally resemble dentine are subdivided into three types depending on their position. The stones which are located in pulp, surrounded by pulp are free uplp stones. There are few pulp stones placed close to dentine on one side and surrounded by pulp on the other three sides are called attached pulp stones.

There is possibility of pulp stones get entrapped into dentine and surrounded by dentine on all sides are called embedded true pulp stones.

Q33. What are the false pulp stones ?
Ans. False pulp stones are composed of masses of classified material which do not exhibit tubular structure. Instead these are made up of concentric layer of calcification around central nidus. The nature of nidus is not clear. However it is believed to be made up of cells and reticular fibers. The false denticles are larger than true denticles and are more often seen in coronal pulp than in radicular pulp.
Like true pulp stones, the false pulp stones are also subdivided into free, attached and embedded (Interstital, depending on their placement).

Q34. Describe diffuse calcification.
Ans. Diffuse calcification is seen in radicular pulp. The calfication occurs along with the degenerated blood vessels. The usual pattern is amorphous, linear calcifications along with the blood vessels.

Q35. What are the clinical features of pulp stones ?
Ans. Most often the pulp stones are asymptomatic, even though few reports had associated pulp stones with severe pain in the tooth. Presence of pulp stones in general neither causes pain nor impinge on nerves.

Q36. Can pulp stones be diagnosed clinically ?
Ans. No. There presence does not cause any typical features.

Q37. How to diagnose pulp stones ?
Ans. Pulp stones are visible as radiopaque structures in radiographs.

Q38. What is the clinical significance of pulp of pulp stones ?
Ans. Pulp stones are most often seen in older teeth Large pulp stones may interfere with the endodontics treatment.

Q39. What is chronic perforating hyperplasia of pulp ?
Ans. Chronic perforating hyperplasia is associated with internal resorption of dentine. It is an idiopathic condition. However trauma seems to be triggering factor in most of the cases. The resorption of dentine on pulpal surface is associated with inflammatory hyperplasia of pulp. The resorption of dentine may case perforation.

Q40. What are the other names of internal resorption of dentine ?
Ans. Idiopathic internal resorption of dentine is also referred to as pink tooth of Mummery, internal granuloma, odontoclastoma and chronic perforating hyperplasia of pulp.

Q41. What are the findings of vitality tests in pink tooth of Mummery ?
Ans. The pink tooth is vital. The vitality tests do not show much significant changes than normal counter part tooth.

Q42. What are the clinical features of pink tooth ?
Ans. Teeth with internal resorption of dentine are invariably asymptomatic. The earliest clinical finding may be appearance of pinkish hue in coronal part. This is due to resorption of dentine and appearance of vascular pulp tissue through translucent enamel. Most often maxillary anterior teeth are affected.

Q43. What are the radiologic appearance in intenal resorption of dentine ?
Ans. In routine radiographs taken, the radiographic finding of internal resorption of dentine may be the first evidence of presence of abnormality. The affected tooth exhibits oval or round radiolucent area on inner walls of dentine and in association with pulpal radioluceny.

Q44. Write the histoloic appearance of idiopathic internal resorption of dentine.

Ans. Microscopic examination of internal resorption shows variable degree of resorption of pulpal end of dentine and proliferation of pulp to fill up the resorbed area, odontoclasts appear in resorbed surface and pulp exhibits chronic inflammatory changes. On few occasions there may be alternating periods of resorption of dentine and formation of new dentine.

Q45. What is the etiology of acute apical periodontitis ?

Ans. Acute apical periodontitis may result as a sequelae of pulpal disease or due to trauma to the tooth. Acute apical periodontitis may also be caused by occlusal overfillings causing occlusal trauma. This will result mostly within first twenty four hours of amalgam fillings.

Q46. Write clinical features of acute apical periodontitis.

Ans. Pain is most prominent feature of acute apical periodontitis. Tooth is severely tender to percussion. Feeling of extension of tooth from socket and premature contact of tooth on occlusion is common feeling. Continuous, severe and radiating type of pain is a common finding.

Q47. What is the etiology of apical granuloma ?

Ans. Apical granuloma is caused as a sequelae of necrotic or gangrenous pulp. It is a mass of granulation tissue formed at apex to wall of the irritants entering the periapical area.

Q48. Write the clinical features of periapical granuloma.

Ans. Periapical granuloma seldom presents with clinical features. It is mostly asymptomatic. However in its initial period of formation, when the pulpal irritants enter the periapical area and cause inflammatory reaction, the clinical features may simulate chronic apical periodontitis. Dull pain, tenderness of tooth, and pain on biting may be observed.

However one may notice discharging fistulous tract in previously exacerbated granuloma leading to abscess formation, perforation of bone and ovelying mucosa, discharging the pus. The tract may remain even after suppuration is cured and abscess Is reverted back to periapical granuloma.

Q49. Describe the radiologic appearance of periapical granuloma.
Ans. In a radiograph, apical granuloma appears as well circumscribed radiolucent area at the apex of the root. The borders of radiolucency arecontinuous with lamina dura. The radiolucency may or may not show cortication. It measures less than 1 cm in diameter. Periapical granuloma with exacerbation or which is expanding may present with diffuse margins in radiogram.

Q50. Describe the histologic feature of periapical granuloma.
Ans. In initial period there is edema of periodontal ligament and infiltration of chronic inflammatory cells. Inflammation and increased vascularity is associated with resorption of adjacent bone. IT is followed by proliferation of fibroblasts and endothelial cells and the formation of more tiny vascular channels, as well as numerous delicate connective tissue fibrils. The new capillaries are usually lined by swollen endothelial cells. The gramuloma is composed predominantly of macrophages, lymphocytes, and plasma cells. The other important finding is presence of epithelium. This is believed to be originating from cell rests of Malazzez. The connective tissue is limited to periphery forming a capsule of condensed bundles of collagen fibres. This is more prominent in slow growing granulomas.

Q51. What is pulse granuloma
Ans. Periapical granuloma sometimes exhibit a peculiar feature of fiant cell hyaline angiopathy, which consists of inflammatory cell infiltration, collection of foreign body type giant cells, presence of ringlike structures composed of eosinophillic material and fragments of foreign material ,sometimes resembling vegetable matter such as legumes and trismus. Firm inflammatory swelling is seen in

preauricular region. Thus the term pulse granuloma is given to such granulomas.

Q52. What is the sequelae of periapical granuloma ?
Ans. Periapical granuloma may form abscess or may give rise to periapical cyst.

Q53. What is periapical abscess ?
Ans. Periapical abscess is a suppurative process of periapical region of tooth, caused most often as sequelae of pulpal diseases. The infection of periapical region may also occur due to traumatic injuries as wel as due to hematogenous source. Infection of periapical ranuloma and cyst may also lead to form an abscess. The periapical abscess can be either acute or chronic.

Q54. Write clinical features of an acute periapical abscess.
Ans. Acute periapical abscess is associated most often with a damaged tooth due to caries, trauma, attrition, abrasion, or erosion. The onset is sudden. Severe and radiating pain is common feature. Pain is aggravated on biting or cheing process. The associated tooth is severely tender. The patient feels that tooth is slightly extruded from socket. Tenderness of tooth as well as alveolar region either on buccal or lingual aspect may be elicited. Regional lymphadenitis is a common finding.

Q55. What are the sequelae of acute periapical abscess ?
Ans. Suppuration in acute periapical abscess may regress due to treatment. In sever cases, the pus may spread to neighbouring structures perforating the bone, thus causing various forms of abscess including subperiosteal, alveolar and cellulites involving more than one facial spaces. An acute periapical abscess may turn into chronic abscess.

Q56. What are the radiological features of acute periapical abscess ?
Ans. Radiographs may not show any significant bony changes in an acute periapical abscess as the suppuration in acute

phase does not cause enough demineralization to produce significant shadows in radiographs. The radiological changes may be evident after about four to six days. In such cases radiolucent area with diffuse margins may b seen in relation to affected apex. Lamina dura gets dissolved therefore discontinuation of lamina dura is evident.

Q57. What are the clinical features of chronic periapical abscess ?
Ans. The clinical sign and symptoms in chronic periapical abscess are less severe than as seen in anacute form. This is due to localization of suppuration to well circumscribed area without an pressure. Tooth is slightly tender. rEgional lymphadenitis is present.

Q58. Write clinical features of subperiosteal abscess.
Ans. Subperiosteal abcess is very painful condition due to collection of pus below the periosteum. Swelling is firm and severely tender. It is seen intraorally in alveolar region in relation to affected tooth.

Q59. Write clinical features of acute Dento-alveolar abscess.
Ans. Dento-alveolar abscess is an odontogenic abscess in which the suppuration has escaped into alveolar mucosal area and loose connective tissue fascia. It is seen as acute swelling which is painful. The swelling is firm, warm and tender. The location swelling depends on the tooth involved and location of suppuration in related fascial spaces, regional lymphadenitis is common feature.

Q60. Which factors determine the route of spread of odontogenic infection ?
Ans. Pus spreads in a least resistant direction. Pus from apical area may traverse either buccally or lingually depending on the proximity of root. The pus perforates bone to spread into soft tissue. Periapical abscess from mandibular last molar usually perforates lingual plate.

Q61. Name the fascial spaces in floor of mouth.
Ans. The fascial spaces located in floor of mouth are submental, sublingual and submandibular fascial spaces.

Q62. What is Ludwig's angina ?
Ans. Ludwig's angina is severe and extensive cellulites involving at the fascial spaces of floor of mouth. It involves spaces of both sides. The spaces involved are submental, sublingual, and submandibular.

Q63. What is the etiology of Ludwig's angina ?
Ans. The periapical, periodontal or pericoronal infection from mandibular third molar is most often responsible for Ludwig's angina. However this may also be caused by injuries of floor of mouth thus infecting the fascial spaces. Even the periapical and periodontal infection from mandibular second molar may also lead to Ludwig's angina. Compound fractures of mandible may also lead to Ludwig's angina.

Q64. Name the fascial spaces which may be involved from the infection of mandibular last molar.
Ans. The varios fascial spaces to which the infection from mandibular last molar can spread include submasseteric, parotid fascial space, pterygomandibular space, fascial spaces of floor of mouth, parapharyngeal and retropharyngeal spaces.

Q65. Write clinical features of Ludwig's angina.
Ans. Ludwig's angina is a severe form of cellulites of floor of mouth. The clinical features include rapidly developing board like swelling of the floor of mouth, elevation of tongue, restricted movements of mandible, difficulty in swallowing as well as breathing, swelling is tender and brawny. General constitutional symptoms include pyrexia, malaise, rapid pulse and rapid respiration. As the infection spreads, it may involve paraphryngeal spaces causing spread of swelling to neck and edema of larynx leading to death due to suffocation. Regional lymphadenitis is common associated finding.

Q66. Write managemtn of LUdig's angina.
Ans. Draingage and administration of antibiotics are prime important. The advancement of antibiotics had considerably reduced the incidence of Ludwig's angina.

Q67. What is phlegmon ?
Ans. Cellulitis is also called phelgmon. Cellulitis, is a diffuse inflammation of soft tissues not restricted to one area but involve fascial spaces.

Q68. Which organisms are associated with cellulites ?
Ans. Cellulitis is caused by organisms that produce enzymes which dissolve intercellular round substance thus enabling rapid spread of infection. The enzymes include hyaluronidase and fibrinolysin Streptococci are particularly potent which produce hyaluronidase enzyme.

Q69. What is the spreading factor of Duran-Reynals ?
Ans. Hyaluronidase, an enzyme which dissolves hyaluronic acid is referred to as spreading factor of duran-Reynals.

Q70. What is fascial space ?
Ans. Fascial space is a space that is present in the soft tissue along with the plane of fascia separating the muscles and other structures. These are potential spaces through which the infection can spread easily.

Q71. Mention few fascial spaces which may be involved by odontogenic infection.
Ans. Submental, sublingual, submandibular, pterylgomandibular, submasseteric, parotid, buccal, infratemporal, lateral pharyngeal, retropharyngeal space and carotid sheath space.

Q72. What are the boundaries of infratemporal fascial space ?

Ans. Infratemporal fascial space is bounded anteriorly by maxillary tuberosity, posteriorly by lateral ptreygoid muscle, coronoid process and temporal muscle. Laterally it is bound by zygomatic arches, tendon of temporalis muscle and origin of masseter muscle. Medially it is bound by lateral terygoid plates and lateral pterygoid muscle. Infratemporal space is situated below the temporal bone. Inferioryly it is continuous with pterygomandibular space.

Q73. What is the location of submasseteric space ?

Ans. Submasseteric space is located between the maseter muscle and lateral surface of mandible. Masseter muscle is attached by three heads.

Q74. Write clinical features of submasseteric abscess.

Ans. Infection from mandibular third molar spreads to submasseteric space. This space also may be involved from the infection of second molar. But this is not common. The patients with submasseteric abscess suffer from sever pain.

Q75. What are the boundaries of submandibular space ?

Ans. Submandibular space is situated in the floor of oral cavity. It is located posteriorly below the mylohyoid muscel. It is bordered medially by hyoglossus muscle and diasttic muscle and laterally by the inner surface of mandible. The space encloses submandibular salivary gland and lymph nodes.

Q76. What are the boundaries of sublingual fascial space ?

Ans. Sublingual fascial space is located anteriorly and superficially. It is bordered inferiorly by mylohyoid muscle, superiorly by mucosa of floor of oral cavity, laterally by the inner aspect of mandible, medially by median raphe of tongue and posteriorly by hyoid bone.

Q77. What is the location of lateral pharyngeal space ?
Ans. The lateral pharyngeal space is one of parapharyngeal spaces. It is located lateral to pharynx and is bounded anteriorly by the buccopharyneal aponeurosis, medical pterygoid muscle, posteriorly by prevertebral fascia, medially by later wall of pharynx and laterally by the carotid sheath.

Q78. What are the boundaries of retropharyngeal space ?
Ans. The retropharyngeal space is located behind pharynx hence anteriorly it is bounded by the posterior wall of pharynx, posteriorly by the prevertebral fascia, laterally by the lateral pharyngeal space and carotid sheath.

Q79. What ar the intracranial complications of odontogenic infection ?
Ans. Variety of intracranial complications have been reported as originating from odontoenic infections. These include cavernous sinus thrombosis, brain abscess, leptomeningitis, subdural empyema and suppurative encephalitis.

Q80. What is osteomyelitis ?
Ans. Osteomyelitis is an inflammation of bone and bone marrow.

Q81. What is the etiology of osteomyelitis ?
Ans. There are various etiological cause of osteomyelitis of jaw bones. Most common being the infection. This could either be o odontogenic in origin or non-odontogenic origin. The other etioloical factors include injuries.

Q82. Which organisms cause osteomyelitis ?
Ans. Osteomylitis of jaws may either be caused by nonspecific organisms (mixed infection) or by the specific organisms like tuberculosis, symphlis, and sctinomycosis.

Q83. Classify the osteomyelitis of jaw bones.

Ans. Osteomyelitis of jaw bones is classified mainly as suppurative and nonsuppurative. Both the groups have acute, subacute and chronic forms.

    I.   Suppurative
        (a) nonspecific   1. Acute   2. Chronic
        (b) Specific   1. Tuberculosis 2. Syphilis
        3. Actinomycosis
    II.   Nonsuppurative
        (a) Sclerosing   1. Focal   2. Diffuse
        (b) Proliferative
        (c) Chemical (phosphorus)
        (d) Osteoradionecrosis.

Q84. What is the etiology of acute suppurative osteomyelitis ?

Ans. Acute suppurative osteomyelitis is most often caused as sequelae of periapical infection. The infection may also be caused by fractures of jaw bones and other injuries. The organisms associated with this form of osteomyelitis are nonspecific like staphylococcus aureus, staphylococcus ablus and streptococcus.

Q85. Write clinical features of acute suppurative osteomyelitis of infants.

Ans. Before the advancement of antibiotic a peculiar form of acute suppurative osteomyelitis of maxilla in infant, and young children was a common finding. The onset is sudden and is associated with inflamed painful swelling in maxilla. Suppuration is a common feature. Pyrexia and malaise are other finding.s This need not be associated with odontogenic infection but most often reported to occur due to hematogenous infection or from minor oral injuries. The acute suppurative osteomylitis of infants had become considerably rare due to availability of better antibiotics.

Q86. Write the clinical features of acute suppurative osteomyelitis.

Ans. Acute suppurative osteomyelitis of jaw bones often results from diffuse spread of infection throughout medullary spaces, with subsequent necrosis of bone. Therefore initial clinical features resemble to that of a dentoalveolar abscess. This may involve either of the jaw bones. In maxilla, the disease tends to be more localized whereas in mandible, it tends to be diffuse. The clinicalfeatures include swelling, severe pain, loosening of related teeth. Which become severely tender. Elevation of temperature and regional lymphadenitis are common features. Paresthesia or anaesthesia of lower lip may present in osteomyelitis of mandible.

Q87. Write histologic features of acute suppurative osteomyelitis.

Ans. Medullary spaces are filled with inflammatory exudates. The inflammatory cells, chiefly polymorphonuclear leukocytes and lymphocytes are found in large umber. The pus may form. Osteoblasts bordering the bony trabeculae get destroyed. The trabecula may loose viability and tend to get resorbed.

Q88. Write radiological features of acute suppurative soteomyelitis.

Ans. There are no specific or diagnostic radiological features in acute phase. There may be evidence of preexisting conditions if any, such as periapical granuloma, cyst or chronic abscess. Acute suppurative osteomyelitis might have resulted from exacerbation of such preexisting conditions.

Radiological changes occur after about a week. The appearance then includes diffuse radiolucency and widening of marrow spaces.

Q89. What is sequestrum ?
Ans. The sequestrum is the separation of dead bone or necrosed bone. Sequestra are common finding in osteomyelitis.

Q90. What is involucrum ?
Ans. The involucrum is the formation of new bone around sequestrum.

Q91. What are the complications of osteomyelitis ?
Ans. Formation of discharging sinuses through wihci sequestrum get discharged, pathologic fractures of bones may occur. Asymmetry of face due to periodtitis and malunion may result.

Q92. What is the management of acute suppurative osteomyelitis ?
Ans. Management of acute suppurative osteomyelitis includes proper drainage of pus, and removal of sequestra if present. Administration of antibiotics and analgesics form an essential part of the management.

Q93. Write the clinical features of chronic suppurative osteomyelitis.
Ans. Chronic suppurative osteomyelitis may result as sequelae of acute phase or may result directly form the infection without any evidence of acute phase. The clinical features are milder than seen in acute phase. However extensive involvement may be seen. Swelling with discharging fistula are common finding. Small pieces of sequestra may get discharged.

Q94. What is condensing osteitis ?
Ans. Condensing osteitis is an unusual response of bone, occurring in instances of extremely high tissue response or in cases of low grade infection.

Q95. Mention the types of condensing osteitis.
Ans. The condensing osteitis could be seen in local form (focal sclerosing osteomyelitis) or in diffuse form involving a wider area of jaw bones.

Q96. Describe the radiographic appearance of focal condensing osteits.
Ans. In the radiographs the focal condensing osteitis appears as well circumscribed radiopaque area at the apex of root or roots. Entire root outline is almost always clearly visible.

Q97. In periapical radiographs which other diseases resemble focal condensing osteitis ?
Ans. Mature cementoma, hypercementosis and florid osseous dysplasia.

Q98. Radiographically how to differentiate between condensing osteitis and other similarly appearing lesions ?
Ans. In addition to clinical feature which may aid in differentiating such lesions from each other radiographically focal condensing osteitis may be differentiated from cementoma from the fact that clear outline of root is visible in condensing osteitis indicating that it is a response of bone. Peridontal space shadow may be visible around the root. This may be absent in cementoma or hypercementosis. In these to, radiopaque shadow is associated with root surface.

Q99. What is Garre's osteomyelitis ?
Ans. Garre's osteomyelitis is an another unusual form of chronic osteomyelitis in which there is proliferative reaction. It was described by Garre in 1893.

Q100. What are the other names of Garre's osteomy elitis?

Ans. Garre's osteomyelitis is also referred as nonsuppurative sclerosing osteitis, chronic proliferative periostitis, and periostitis ossificans.

Q101. Write clinical features of Garre's osteomyelitis.

Ans. It is seen in children and young adults and more common in mandible than in maxilla. The patient may present with history of mild pain of long duration. Bony hard diffuse swelling may be present usually on outer surface of body of mandible, in relation to carious or infected tooth.

Q102. Describe radiographic appearance of Garre's osteomyelitis.

Ans. The changes in periapical radiograph are not much significant except that the evidence carious tooth and periapical rarefaction may be present. Howeverthe occlsal radiographs show typical oniorpeel appearance sescribed as duplication of cortication. This represents well formed smooth layers of ossification.

7.

INJURIES OF ORAL CAVITY: REPAIR AND ALTERATION OF THE TEETH

Q1. What are the causes of tooth fracture ?
Ans. The most frequent cause of fracture of teeth is severe and sudden trauma. Trauma may result from fall, automobile accident, assault and injuries associated with games and sports. Latrogenic causes include accidental trauma of neighboring teeth while undertaking extraction of other teeth. Teeth with large restorations, root canal fillings, large carious lesions, internal resorption, severe cervical abrasion and with faulty restoration are likely to be fractured due to masticatory forces.

Q2. Which are the teeth, more prone for fractures ?
Ans. Maxillary anterior and mandibular anterior teeth are more likely to get fractured.

Q3. Which factors influence the most in treatment of fracture of teeth ?
Ans. The very important and significant factor which modifies the treatment plan is intactness of pulp or involvement of pulp.

Q4. How the injuries of teeth classified ?
Ans. Injuries of teeth are classified according to Elli's classification.

Q5. Elli's classification composed of how many groups ?
Ans. Elli's calssified the injuries of teeth into nine groups.

Q6. Classify the injuries of the deciduous teeth.
Ans. The injuries of the deciduous teeth are classified as class IX of Ellis classification.

Q7. Classify the injuries of teeth according to Elli's classification.
Ans. The injuries of teeth are classified into nine groups under Elli's classification class I is somple fracture of teeth involving little or no dentine. Class-II consists of extensive fracture of crown involving considerable dentine but not the pulp. Class-III injuries consists of extensive fracture involving enamel, dentine and pulp. In Class IV the traumatized tooth becomes nonvital. Class V injuries are those in which tooth is lost. Traumatised tooth with fracture of roots is classified as class VI. Displacement of tooth with or without fracture of crown or root is classified as class VII. Fracture of crown en mass and its replacement is classified into class VIII. Injuries to the deciduous teeth are grouped into class IX.

Q8. What are the causes of maxillofacial injuries ?
Ans. Most of the maxillofacial injuries are caused by road transport accident. The other causes include injuries from fall, games physical injuries caused in fights and assaults, injuries related to occupation and industries, injuries caused by weapons like clubs, knives and fire arms.

Q9. What type of primary care is required in maxillofacial injuries ?
Ans. Every patient with maxillofacial injuries shall be examined carefully and in detail for intracranial involvement, blockage of airway and hemorrhage. Primary care includes removal of air way blockage, maintenance of airway, control of hemorrhage and restoration of fluid loss.

Q10. Name the different mechanical wounds of soft tissues ?
Ans. Contusion, abrasion, lacerations incised wounds, stab wounds, fire arm wounds, dislocations and fractures are the different forms of injuries of wounds.

Q11. What is incised wound ?
Ans. Incised wound is a clean cut through the tissues. It is caused by sharp cutting edged devise like knife, scalpel, sword etc.

Q12. What is lacerated injury ?
Ans. Lacerations are tears or splits of skin or mucosa by application of blunt force to the broad area of tissues. The tissues are destroyed. The margins of wounds are well separated and irregular.

Q13. What is abrasive injury ?
Ans. Abrasive wounds are partial loss of superficial layers of epithelium. These are caused by fall on rough surface or being dragged during fall. Abrasive wounds are painful and irregular in shape.

Q14. What is contusion wounds ?
Ans. A contusion wound is an effusion of blood onto the tissue due to rupture of blood vessels caused by blunt trauma. It may occur not only on skin but also on internal organs.

Q15. What is ecchymosis ?
Ans. Ecchymosis is bleeding from ruptured blood vessels in the superficial layer of subepithelium.

Q16. Which are the weak areas of mandible which are prone for fracture ?
Ans. The area occupied by more amount of tooth substance, the area having foramen or thin bony area. Hence the canine area, molar area, angle of mandible and subcondylar areas are more prone for fractures.

Q17. Classify fractures of bone.
Ans. Bone fractures can be classified in many ways. Fracture is said to be direct if the fracture occurs at the site of impact and indirect if the fracture. Occurs away from the site of impact. Fractures can also be classified depending on the fragments. Simple fracture is the fracture in which

overlying tissues are intact and fragments of bone are not exposed to exterior. The greenstick fractures are those in whichfracture is incomplete or only one cortex of bone is fractured.

The comminuted fractures are those in which the bone fractures into multiple fragments. The compound fracture is the fracture in which the fractured bone is exposed to exterior.

Q18. What is favourable fracture ?
Ans. Fracturs in which the fragments resist the pull of muscles and are not displaced are called favourable fractures. In such cases the direction of muscle pull is at right angle to the fracture line.

Q19. What is unfavorable fracture ?
Ans. The fractures in which the muscle pull cause the displacement of fracments.

Q20. What are the different wounds encountered in oral cavity ?
Ans. Extraction woulnds, biopsy wounds, soft tissue wounds and fracture of jaw bones are the few common wounds in oral cavity.

Q21. How do the wounds of oral cavity differ from extra oral wounds ?
Ans. The unusual anatomic situations of oral cavity makes it differ in certain aspects. The presence of teeth surrounded by giniva which often remains inflamed, the presence of different microorganisms in warm, and moist dedium of saliva and difficulty in applying closed dressings are the factors which contribute to modify the healing process. The difficulty in immobilizing the part like jaw bones and angle of mouth also contribute in delayed healing. However warmth of oral cavity may accelerate the wound healing.

Q22. What are the the factors which may influence the healing of oral wounds ?

Ans. The factors which influence the would healing include physical factors, circulatory factors, nutritional factors, hormonal factors, age, infections and location of wounds.

Q23. What are the physical factors which influence the wound healing ?

Ans. Severity of trauma or injury is an important factor as simple and small wounds heal early. Severely damaged tissue may take long time. The second wound inflicted in a site of healing initial wound, heals more rapidly than the initial wound. Local temperature (hyperthermia) also accelerates the healing.

Q24. What are the circulatory factors which influence the wound healing ?

Ans. Wounds in area in which there is rich cascular bed heal more rapidly than in avascular area. Anemia may delay healing. Dehydration may also delay the healing process.

Q25. What are the nutritional factors which influence the wound healing ?

Ans. The wound healing may be influenced by many nutritional factors. Protein is an important constituent of food which influence wound healing. Protein is essential for rapid healing. Vitamins are also important factors for rapid wound healing. Vitamin C (Ascorbic Acid) is essential for collagen formation and ground substance of connective tissue. The deficiency of other vitamins like A, D and B complex may also delay the wound healing.

Q26. What are the types of healing of Biopsy wounds ?

Ans. Biopsy wound healing can either be primary or secondary healing.

Q27. What is primary healing ?

Ans. Primary healing is the healing is the healing of wounds in which the edges are brought together into apposition often by suturing. It is also referred to as healing by primary intension or healing by first intention.

Q28. Described the primary healing.
Ans. When the edges of the wound are brought together and held in place by sutures, the blood clots and numerous leukocytes are mobilized into the area. Connective tissue cells in the area undergo transformation into fibroblasts. The fibroblasts multiply rapidly and beigin to migrate in and around the wound. In due course, these cells form thin, delicate collagen fibrils, which intertwine and coalesce in a general direction parallel to the surface of the wound. Endothelial cells proliferate forming thin new capillaries, which are filled with blood. When the edges of the wound are in close apposition epithelium proliferates rapidly closing the wounds.

Q29. What is secondary healing ?
Ans. Secondary healing is the healing of open wounds. It is also called as healing by granulation, and healing by second intention.

Q30. Describe the mechanism of secondary healing.
Ans. The secondary healing occurs in wounds in which the edges cannot be approximated due to loss of tissue. The loss of tissue is replaced from granulation tissue. The wound is filled with blood which clots. The proliferation of fibroblasts and endothelial cells is slow. Cellular proliferation begins at periphery and fills up the complete wounds. Polymorphonuclear leukocytes and later lymphocytes and mononuclear phagocytes migrate to granulation tissue. As the granulation tissue matures, it becomes more fibrous and surface becomes epithelized.

Q31. What are the immediate reactions in the tooth socet after extraction of tooth ?
Ans. The blood which fills the socket coagulates and forms a clot. Red blood cells being entrapped in fibrin mesh work. First few hours of blood clot are critical. It is likely to be dislodged resulting in delayed and painful healing. Initial

changes in the healing socket include vasodilatation and engorgement of remnants of blood vessels in periodontal ligament. The clot is covered by thick layer of fibrin. Gingiva around the socket collapses, partly covering the socket opening.

Q32. What is the average time taken for healing of socket after tooth extraction ?
Ans. Healing of socket after extraction of tooth may occur between 4 to 6 weeks.

Q33. What are the changes occurring during first week of healing of tooth socket ?
Ans. After the clot has settled, the proliferation of fibroblasts from connective tiseue cells in the remember nants of periodontal ligament is evident. The fibroblasts begin to grow into clot. The blood clot acts as a scaffold upon which the cells associated with the healing process may migrate. Osteoclasstic activity becomes evident at crest of alveolar bone. Endothelial cells start proliferating. There is no evidence of formation of osteoid tissue.

Q34. Write the changes occurring during second week of healing of socket.
Ans. During the second week healing, the fibroblast multiply at rapid rate and grow into the clot which appears as fibrinous mesh work. New delicate capillaries form and penetrate to center of clot. The remnants of periodontal ligament undergo degeneration. Alveolar socket shows marked osteoclastic activity. Osteoid tissue may appear extending from the walls of socket. In smaller socket epithelization may occur.

Q35. What are the changes seen during third week of healing of socket ?
Ans. During the third week of healing the clot appears organized by maturing granulation tissue. Trabeculae of osteoid bone are forming aound the whole of the socket. The osteoblasts originate from the pluripotent cells of remnants of periodontal ligament. Alveolar crest becomes

small and rounded off due to osteoclastic resorption. The socket well also gets partly resorbed and appears less dense. Epithelization may occur.

Q36. What are the final changes occurring in the healing of socket ?
Ans. Filling of socket with bone and remodeling of bone occur in final stages occurring in fourth week. Maturation of bone may continue even upto 6 to 8 weeks. As the alveolar crest undergoes resorption, the crest of healed socket is at lower level than neighboring area.

Q37. What is the radiographic appearance of healed socket in fourth week ?
Ans. Even though bone filling occurs in fourth week after extraction, bone is not calcified fully, hence the socket appears slightly radiolucent than neighboring bone.

Q38. What is dry socket ?
Ans. Dry socket is complication occurring during healing of socket. It is also called as alveolitis siccadolorosa, and alveolar osteitis. It is a form of focal osteomyelitis.

Q39. What are the causes of dry socket ?
Ans. Dry socket is mostly associated with difficult or traumatic extractions.
Dislodgment of clot is the basic mechanism in production of dry socket. The clot may be dislodged due to various causes including smoking, consumption of fluids and food within few hours of extraction. Infection may occur easily in empty socket.

Q40. Write clinical features of dry socket.
Ans. Sockets of mandibular molars are prone for dry socket. Dry ocket usually occurs after first tow or three days. But may also occur later. The condition develops as a severely painful condition after 2 or 3 days. Foul smell is common but there is no suppuration. Socket appears empty. Necrosis of bone fragment may occur.

Q41. Write the management of dry socket.
Ans. The dry socet is extremely painful and healing is delayed. Management of dry socket includes reduction of pain and promotion of healing. Local dressing with obtundent, antibacterial paste are advocated for local use.

Q42. What is myospherulosis ?
Ans. Myospherulosis is a complication of healing of an extaction or soft tissue wound into which there has been placed antibiotic ointment with petrolatum base. This results in the formation of clear spaces within the area of healing and presence of altered erythrocytes which resemble clusters of spherules. This appearance is mistaken for large microorganism.

Q43. What is the initial change in fractures of bone ?
Ans. Initial change in fracture of bones is cutting or tearing of blood vessels, extravasation of blood and loss of blood supply to the proximal end. The blood clot plays an important but passive role in healing fractures. Granulation tissue replaces blood clot and subsequently callus forms.

Q44. What is callus ?
Ans. The callus is the structure which unites the fracture ends of bones and it is composed of varying amounts of fibrous tissue, cartilage and bone.

Q45. Write the mechanism of formation of callus ?
Ans. The periosteum is an important and essential part in the formation of callus. The cells of periosteum near fracture ends die but cells peripheral to that proliferate. These cells assume the feature and activity of osteoblasts. The continuous proliferation of these cell forms a collar of callus. The differentiation of cells into osteoblasts and subsequent formation of bone occure in the deepest part of callus collar. Little away from the fracture line, cells differentiate into chondrocytes instead of osteoblasts and lay down cartilage.

Q46. What is the amount cartilage in callus ?
Ans. The amount of cartilage formed in a callus varies remarkably in different areas and the amount is determined by several factors.

Q47. What are the factors influencing the formation of cartilage ?
Ans. The factors influencing the formation of cartilage includes vascularity, speed of healing process and movement of fragments of fractured bone. In well vascularised environment bone formation is predominant and cartilage is poorly formed. In less vascularised areas cartilage formation is more. In slowly healing fractures cartilage formation is minimal . In poorly immobilized fractures or moving fracture ends, the amount of cartilage formed is more when compared to fractures well immobilized.

Q48. What are the types of callus ?
Ans. There are internal and external callus. Internal callus forms from the endosteum of haversian canals, and undifferentiated cellws of the bone marrow. The external callus forms from the subperiosteal osteoblasts.

Q49. What are the complications of fracture ?
Ans. The complications includes osteomyelitis, malunion, nonunion and fibrous union.

Q50. What is non union ?
Ans. Nonunion is complication of healing process wherein calluses formed over each fragment fail to meet in fracture line or endosteal formation of bone is inadequate.

Q51. What is malunion ?
Ans. Malunion is occasional complication occurring when fragment are maligned and healing occurs resulting in malposition or malformation.

Q52. What is fibrous union ?
Ans. Fibrous union in fractures is another complication of healing which arise usually as a result of lack of proper

immobilization or fixation of fracture bone. The fractured ends are united by fibrous tissue and there is failure of ossification.

Q53. What are the causes for injury to the pulp tissue ?
Ans. Pulp tissue may be injured in various way. Dental caries may itself cause some damages. Sudden trauma to the tooth may cause injury to pulp. Restorative procedures like cavity preparation, crown reduction, cavity dressing, cavity drying and cavity filling materials may cause damage to pulp tissue.

Q54. Which factors in tooth cutting may influence pulpal injury ?
Ans. Thermal changes during tooth cutting is a major factor which may influence pulpal changes.

Q55. Which factors influence the heat production during tooth cutting ?
Ans. Theremal changes or heat production is influenced by size, shape and composition of bur or stone, speed of bur or stone, direction and amount of pressure on the cutting instrument, length of time the bur or stone in contact with the tooth surface and the amount of moisture in the field of operation and finally the type of tissue being cut (enamel or dentine).

Q56. How do the filling material cause the pulpal injury ?
Ans. The filling materials may cause pulpal injury by production of heat during setting process or y contents of acid.

Q57. Which are the chemicals which may cause tissue damage ?
Ans. Local application of aspirin causes chemical burn of superficial tissueof mucosa. This is known as aspirin burn. Local application on mucosa of eugenol, phenol, trichloroacetic acid, silver nitrate, Zinc chloride and concentrate hydrogen peroxide may also cause soft tissue injuries. Acrylic may also cause tissue damage in certain individuals.

Q58. What are the soft tissue injury caused by dentures?
Ans. Traumatic ulcer, hyperplasia of tissue and papillary hyperplasia of palatal mucosa may be caused by dentures.

Q59. What is Epulis fissuratum ?
Ans. Epulis fissuratum is hyperplasia of oral mucosa around the over extended flanges of dentures. There are painless growth and correspond to the border of denture.

Q60. What is Inflammatory papillary hyperplasia ?
Ans. Inflammatory papillary hyperplasia is an inflammatory reaction seen in denture wearers. It is most often seen in those who wear denture continuously through out. The papillary red inflammatory projection are observed on palatal mucosa. These papillary projections appear as thick and warty appearance.

8.

MUCOCUTANEOUS DISORDERS

Q1. Mention diseases which may have oral manifestations and skin abnormalities.

Ans. Ectodermal dysplasia and chondroectodermal dysplasia have manifestations in skin, teeth, hair, bones and nails.

Q2. Name few skin diseases, which may also have mucosal lesion.

Ans. Diseases of skin which also exhibit mucosal lesions are referred to as muco-cutaneous disorders. These include lichen planus, pemphigus, pemphigoid, erythema multiform, eratosis follicularis, epidermolysis bullosa and sclerosis.

Q3. Write the manifestations of ectodermal dysplasia.

Ans. Ectodermal dysplasia is also called hereditary hypohidrotic or anhidrotic ectodermal dysplasia. It is a hereditary condition characterized by congenital dysplasia of one or more structure of ectodermal origin or their appendages. The manifestations include hypohidrosis, hypotrichosis and hypodontia. Various abnormalities like dry skin, thin and spares hair, andontia, absence of sweat glands, depressed nose, and ronounced supraorbital ridges and frontal bossing may be prominent features. The individuals suffer from hyperpyrexia due to absence of seat glands.

Q4. What is the genodermatoses ?

Ans. Term genodermatoses is used to describe certain hereditary skin disorders which are accompanied by various systemic manifestations.

Q5. What is genokeratoses ?
Ans. Genokeratoses are the hereditary skin diseases associated with abnormal keratinization process.

Q6. What is Lichen planus ?
Ans. Lichen panus is a relatively common muco-cuta-neous disease, which may exhibit manifestation either on skin or oral mucosa or on both together.

Q7. Describe the skin lesions seen in lichen planus.
Ans. The skin lesions of lichen planus are mostly constant and are flat violaceous papules with fine thin scales on the surface. These lesions cause itching sensation.

Q8. What is the etiology of lichen planus ?
Ans. Definite etiology of lichen planus is not known. It is most often present in individuals suffering from stress. Etiology also involves cell mediated, immunologic reaction.

Q9. What are the types of lichen planus ?
Ans. Clinically lichen planus is described in different forms. Hypertrophic, bullous, atrophic, erosive and reticular.

Q10. Mention the common sites of skin lesions in lichen planus.
Ans. The skin lesions may occur on any part of skin, however the most common site being flexor surfaces of forearms and srists, inner aspect of knees and thighs and sacral area of trunk. They are bilaterally symmetrical.

Q11. What types of mucosal lesions are seen in lichen planus ?
Ans. Maculopapular erosive lesions are seen in lichen planus.

Q12. Describe the clinical appearance of reticular form of lichen planus.
Ans. The reticular form of lichen planus consists of slightly elevated, fine papules, arranged in lace like lines. The

linear arrangement may appear as radiating lines or annular (ring like). These fine radiating lines are referred to as striae of wickham. Reticular form is the commonest form among all the types of lichen planus. The lesions may be seen on buccal mucosa, tongue and alveolar mucosa and present bilaterally.

Q13. Describe the clinical features of atrophic lichen planus.

Ans. Atrophic forms of lichen planus occurs with less frequency. Clinically it appears as smooth, red, poorly defined areas with peripheral striae. It may be asymptomatic or have burning sensation. Alveolar mucosa, buccal mucosa may be effected.

Q14. What is the location of antigen antibody reaction in lichen palnus.

Ans. Immunofluorescent tests have demonstrated localization of antibody at basement membrane.

Q15. What are the civatte bodies ?

Ans. Civatte bodies are degenerated epithelial cells of phagocytosed epithelial cell remnants within the macrophage. These appear as round eosinophillic globules. Civatte bodies are also known as colloid bodies, hyaline bodies or fibrillar bodies.

Q16. Describe the microscopic features of lichen planues.

Ans. Lichen planus exhibits typical microscopic features. These include hyperparakeratosis or hyperorthokeratosis, thickening of granular layer and acanthosis. Intracellular edema of spinous layer may be present sometimes. Retepeges develop saw tooth appearance. The basal cell layer may show liquefaction degeneration resulting in appearance of thin band of eosinophillic coagulum. Civatte bodies are present in epithelium. Subepithelial layer may show infiltration of inflammatory cells in papillary zone of lamina propria. These inflammatory cells are arranged in band like arrangement.

Q17. Write the management of lichen planus.
Ans. Various forms of managementincluding medications, surgery and cryotherapy have been advocated. Most often the lesion in lichen planus are diffused, hence surgery and cryotherapy may not be accessible. Medical treatemtn includes antihistamines, cortisones and retinoids. These could be mostly used locally either in the form of cream, gel, aerosol spray, or solution. Reticular form may show regression on its own to reappear again. However erosive form most often requires active medication.

Q18. Describe the clinical features of psoriasis.
Ans. In psoriasis, the skin lesions are characterized by small, sharply demarcated dry papules. Each papule is covered by delicate silvery scale. If the scales are removed, one or more tiny bleeding points become visible. This characteristic feature is called Auspitz's sign. Thjese cutaneous lesions appear on various locations, including scalp, back, face, extremities and chest. The disease is severe in writer and may show remission in summer due to exposure to ultraviolet light.

Q19. Write oral manifestations of psoriasis.
Ans. Oral mucosal lesions are uncommon in psoriasis. However few studies have reported of appearance of popular lesions with an erythematous area.

Q20. What is Monro's abscess ?
Ans. Intraepithelial microabscesses seen in psoriasis are known as monor's abscesses.

Q21. Describe Microscopic features of psoriasis.
Ans. Histologic features of psoriasis are characterized by parakeratosis, elongation and clubbing of retepegs. The epithelium over connective tissue papilla is thinned, through which the tortuous capillary loops of papillae appear. This gives appearance of red spots clinically (Auspitz's sign). Mild lymphocytic infiltration in connective tissue is a common finding.

Q22. What is Erythema multiform ?
Ans.   Erythema multiform is an acute dermatologic disease of unknown etiology and exhibiting protean manifestations.

Q23. What is the characteristic feature of Erythema multiform ?
Ans.   Appearance of vesiculobullous lesions and taget lesions are characteristic features of Erythema multiform.

Q24. What is etiology of Erythema multiform ?
Ans.   Definete etiology of Erythema multiform is not known. Hoever various agents are known to precipitate the onset of the disease in few individuals. Some of the cases, the disease appears to occur spontaneously without any specific agent. Various drugs like barbiturates, Phenylbutazone, salicylates, Contrceptive pils are believed to be precipitating agents in certain cases. Viral bacterial and fungal infections may also trigger the onset of Erythema multiform.

Q25. Describe the clinical features of erythema Multiform.
Ans.   Erythema multiform may occur in any age but mostly it is seen young adults and more common In males. The onset may eb spontaneous with development of asymptomatic erythematous macules, papules, vesicles and bullae. These are distributed symmetrically over the hands, arms, feet, legs, face and neck. The lesions may vary in size in different sites in same individual. The lesions on the hands, feet and ankles may present a typical appearance of concentric ring like lesions of varying shades of erythema. These are described as "Target", "Irish" or "Bulls's eye" lesions.

Q26. What are the oral manifestations of Erythema multiform ?
Ans.   There are no specific characteristic lesion of erythema multiform on oral mucosa. The lesions may present in different forms like macule, papule, vesicles or bullae. The vesicles and bullae rupture leaving erosive or ulcerative

lesions, which are painful. Ulcers are covered with crusted blood. The lesions may be present on lips, toungue, palate, buccal mucosa and gingival.

Q27. What is differential diagnosis of Erythema Multiform ?

Ans. Protean clinical features of Erythema multiform may present difficulty in diagnosis. The oral lesions may be differentiated from pemphigus, bullous lichen planus, acute necrostising ulcerative gingivitis and herpes stomatitis.

Q28. Describe the microscopic features of Erythema Multiform.

Ans. Oral mucosal lesion generally exhibit intracellular edema of spinous layer as well as edema of lamina propria, which may produce subepithelial vesicle or bullae. On the other hand other lesions may exhibit severe liquefaction degeneration within the epithelium resulting in intraepithelial vesicle or bullae. Lymphocytic and eosinophilic cell infiltration may be observed below epithelium.

Q29. What is the treatment of Erythema Multiform ?

Ans. Even though there is no specific treatment, the corticorsteroids have been found more effective in treatemtn of Erythema multiform.

Q30. What is Stevens-Johson Syndrome ?

Ans. Stevens-Johnson Syndrome is a severe and acute bullous from of erythema multiform. It involves widespread area and organs. The onset of the disease is sudden with occurrence of fever, malaise, photophobia and eruptions on oral mucosa, genitalia and skin. The vesicles and bullae leave hemorrhagic surfaces. Eye lesions consists of photophobia, conjunctivitis and corneal ulcerations. The genital lesions include nonspecific urethritis, balanitis and vaginal ulcers.

Q31. What is pemphigus ?
Ans. Pemphigus is a serious, and chronic mucocutaneous disease characterized by small vesicles or large bullae.

Q32. Mention the type of Pemphigus.
Ans. Several types of pemphigus have been reported. Four of these are well recognized. These are pemphigus vulgaris, Pemphigus vegetans, pemphigus foliaceous and pemphigus erythematosus.

Q33. What is the basic lesion of all the types of pemphigus ?
Ans. Vesicle or bullae is the basic lesion of all the types of pemphigus.

Q34. Which type of pemphigus usually exhibits oral mucosal lesion ?
Ans. Oral mucosal lesions mostly occur in pemphigus vulgaris and sometimes in pemphigus vegetans.

Q35. Describe the clinical features of pemphigus Vulgaris.
Ans. Pemphigus mostly occurs in age group of over 30 years. The incidence is equal in both the sexes. Pemphigus Vulgaris is characterized by rapid appearance of bullae which enlarge by lateral spread. Initially lesion may occur on skin, over the trunk, arms and neck. Sometimes oral lesions may precede the skin lesions. The bullae which contain tthin fluid may rupture leaving raw eroded areas. The characteristic feature is the positive NIKOLSKY'S sign. Nikolsky's sign is appearance of vesicler or bulla on lateral application of pressure over the skin of mucosa. Wider involvement may prove fatal due to loss of fluid and secondary infection. Sometimes it may show recovery and remission in few weeks.

Q36. Write the clinical features ofpemphigus Veetans.
Ans. Pemphigus Veetans is considered as a variant of pemphigus vulgaris. The bullae rupture and the eroded

area exhibit "Vegetations" These are covered by purulent exudates.

Q37. Write the clinical features of pemphigus foliaceous?
Ans. The oral manifestations in the type of pemphigus are uncommon. The skin lesions characterized by bullous lesions which rapidly rupture and dry leaving flakes and scales.

Q38. Describe the clinical features of pemphigues erythematosus.
Ans. Pemphigus erythematosus is a vesiculo-bullous disease, which is characterized by thin valled bullae, which rpture leaving eroded areas. These areas resemble seborrheic dermatitis or lupus erythematosus.

Q39. What type of bulla is seen in pemphigus ?
Ans. Pemphigus is characterized by bullae, which are intraepithelial. The fluid is collected within the epithelium above basal cell layer. These bullae are described as surabasillar bullae or vesicles.

Q40. What are the tzanck cells ?
Ans. Tzanck cells are acantholytic or degenerative cells which are found in vesicles or bullae in pemphigus. These cells are characterized by degenerative changes which include swelling and hyper-chromatism of the nuclei. There is an increase in RNA in the cytoplasm. The acantholytic cells are produced by prevesicular edema and dissolution of intercellular attachments.

Q41. What is Tzanck test ?
Ans. Tzanck test is process of collection of acantholytic cells from vesicles or bullae and examination under microscope.

Q42. Describe the microscopic features of pemphigus.
Ans. Initially pemphigus is characterized by prevesicular edema and loss of intercellular bridges. Subsequently separation or split of epithelial cells from basal cell layer is seen. The vesicles and bullae are suprabasillar or intraepithelial. Fluid

from bullae contains Tzanck cells, polymorphonuclear leukocytes and lymphocytes. Pemphigus is characterized by absence of inflammatory cell infiltration in connective tissue.

Q43. Write the findings of imminofluorescent tests in pemphigus.
Ans. Direct immunofluorescent tests is used to demonstrate the presence of immunoglobulins in the intercellular spaces or intercellular substance in the epithelium of the lesion or normal epithelium adjacent to the lesion. These immunoglobulins are IgG, IgA or IgM.

Q44. Write the management of pemhius ?
Ans. Management of pemphigus includes topicaland systemic administration of corticosteroids. Antibiotics are used to control secondary infection.

Q45. What in Bengin Mucous membrane pemphigoid ?
Ans. Bengin mucous membrane pemphigoid is a vesiculobullous disease of unknown etiology affecting oral mucosa and eye. It is also known as cicatricial pemphigoid or ocular pemphigus.

Q46. Described the clinical features of cicatricial pemphigoid ?
Ans. The cicatricial pemphigoid occurs in older age group individuals. It affects females more often than mals. Vesiculobullous lesions occur on oral mucosa and ocnjunctiva. These heal by scare formation. Mucous membrane of nose, larynx, pharynx, esophagus, vagina and penis may also be affected on few occasions. These are uncommon site. The most significant is development of adhesions between palpebral and bulbar conjunctivae.

Q47. What is the type of bulla in cicatricial pemphigoid ?
Ans. The bullae and vesicles are subepithelial type in cicatricial pemphigus or benign mucous membrane pemphigoid.

Q48. Write microscopic findings of lesion of cicatricial pemphigoid ?

Ans. The microscopical features are nonspecific. There is no acantholysis. The separations or degeneration occurs at basement membrane below the epithelium. Therefore the vesicles or bullae are sub-epithelial and thick walled. Connective tissue exhibits inflammatory cell infiltration.

Q49. What is the location of antibodies in the lesion of cicatrical pemphigoid ?

Ans. Immunofluorescence studies have shown the presence of tissue bound basement membrane antibodies, Therefore they are seen along with basement membrane.

Q50. What is the differential diagnosis of cicatricial pemphigoid ?

Ans. The various conditions to be considered in differential diagnosis of cicatricial pemphigoid include erythema multiform, bullous lichen planus, pemphigus vulgaris and bullous pemphigoid.

Q51. Which are the drugs useful in the treatment of benin mucous membrane pemphigoid ?

Ans. Topical or systemic corticosteroids are useful in the treaement of benign mucous membrane pemphigoid.

Q52. What is parapemphigus ?

Ans. Parapemphigus or bullous pemphigoid is another vesiculo bullous disease, considered to be variant of dermatitis herpetiformis.

Q53. Write clinical features of parapemphigus ?

Ans. Parapemphigus or bullous pemphigoid is basically a disease of old age group. The skin lesions appear as generalized ash on limbs. It is prurtic. The rash may remain for few weeks before apperacne of vesicl3s and bullae. The vesicles and bullae are thick walled and also occur on abdomen, nec and legs.

Q54. What are the oral manifestations of parapemphigus?

Ans. The oral mucosal lesions in paraemhigous are not very common like either in pemphigus vulgaris or cicatricial pemphigoid. The lesion may be vesicles, bullae or erosive erythematous area. These may be present on gingiva, buccal mucosa.

Q55. What is the type of bulla in parapemphigus ?

Ans. The vesicles or bullae are of sub-epithelial type in parapemphigus. Separation occurs at the junction of epithelium and basement membrane.

Q56. What is epidermolysis Bullosa ?

Ans. Epidermolysis bullosa is an uncommon dermatological disease in which vesiculo-bullous lesion develop spontaneously after a minor trauma. There are different form of the disease.

Q57. Classify Epidermolysis bullosa.

Ans. Epidermolysis bullosa is classified into different forms. They are epidermolysis cullosa simplex, Epidermoysis bullosa dystrophic, Junctional epidermolysis bullosa, and epidermolysis bullosa acquisita.

Q58. Which of the types of epidermolysis bullosa exhibit oral manifestation ?

Ans. Not all the types of epidermolysis bullosa are known to exhibit the oral manifestations. The oral mucosal lesions are more common in epidermolysis bullosa dystrophic.

Q59. What are the oral mucosal lesions of epidermolysis bullosa dystrophic ?

Ans. Bullae occur on the oral mucosa. These bullae are preceded by the appearance of white spots or erythematous areas. The bullae may be initiated by simple, mild injuries or pressure or with even minor dental operative procedure. The bullae rupture leaving ulcers or erosions which are painful. Scare formation may result in obliteration of sulci and restriction of movements of tongue.

Q60. What are the other oral manifestations associated with epidermolysis bullosa dystrophic ?

Ans. In addition to oral mucosal lesions, defects of teeth have been described. These include hypoplastic teeth, missing teeth, rudimentary teeth and teeth denuded of enamel. However these are very uncommon.

Q61. Mention the type of lupus erythematosus.

Ans. Lupus erythematosus is of two types Systemic lupus erythematosus and 2) Discoid lupus erythematosus.

Q62. What is the etiology of the lupus erythematosus ?

Ans. Variety of etiologic factors have been advocated on the causation of lupus erythematosus. These include genetic predisposing, an immunologic abnormality possibly mediated by viral infection.

Q63. Write the clinical features of systemic lupus erythematosus.

Ans. Systemic lupus erythematosus is systemic cutaneous disease exhibiting exacerbations and remissions. It affects females more than males. Age of occurrence is above 40 years. The cutaneous lesions on face consist of erythematous patches which coalesce to form a roughly symmetrical, bilateral distribution over cheeks and ridge of the nose. It is described as butterfly distribution. Such erythematous cutaneous lesions may also occur on neck, arms and shoulders. These may result in burring or aching sensation. In systemic lupus erythematosus, the organ like kidneys, heart and joints are also involved.

Q64. Describe the clinical features of discoid lupus erythematosus.

Ans. Discoid lupus erythematosus is relatively more common than systemic. The mucocutaneous lesions may occur on oral mucosa and skin of chest, back, and extremities. The typical skin lesions are macules that are often covered by thin grey scale, which on removal leave extensions dipped into enlarged pilosebaceous canals. These are described as "Carpet tack". Butterfly distribution of skin lesions over the face may also occur.

Q65. Write the oral manifestations of lupus erythematousus.

Ans. Oral mucous membrane is involved more often in systemic form than discoid form. The oral mucosal lesions in discoid form begin as erythematous areas with white spots. Ulcerations or erosions may be seen. The margins of the lesions are not well demarcated but show white radiating lines. These lesions may occur on buccal, labial and lingual mucosa. The lesions are similar in systemic form but may show more tendency for bleeding and petechiae.

Q66. What is the differential diagnosis of oral mucosal lesions of lupus erythematosus ?

Ans. Various lesions like candidiasis, lichen planus and leukoplakia shall be considered in differential diagnosis of oral mucosal lesions of lupus erythematosus.

Q67. What is CREST syndrome ?

Ans. It is an uncommon variant of systemic sclerosis. It is an acronym of five major findings. These are calcinosis cutis, raynaud's phenomena, Esophageal dysfunction, sclerodacytyly and telangiectasia.

Q68. What is systemic sclerosis ?

Ans. Systemic sclerosis is characterized by progressive fibrosis of the skin and multiple organs. It was earlier known as scleroderma.

Q69. Write the clinical features of systemic sclerosis.

Ans. Systemic sclerosis is a disease exhibiting progressive fibrosis of the skin, and fixation of the epidermis to the underlying deeper subcutaneous tissues. It usually begins on the face, hands or trunk. Neuralgia, paraesthesia and arthritis may develop. Skin may show brown pigmentations. Calcification and hardening of the skin occurs, leading to mask like appearance of face.

Q70. What is morphea ?
Ans. Morphea is a local form of scleroderma. These occur as localized areas of thickening or fibrotic patches of white or yellowish color. These appear irregular in shape and surrounded by violaceous halo.

Q71. Write oral manifestations of systemic sclerosis.
Ans. Progressive sclerosis may involve tongue, soft palate and mucosa. This leads to stiffening of the parts. Sclerosis is preceded by edema of the area. Fibrosis or sclerosis may cause dysphagia, inability to open mouth, and difficult in breathing. Involvement of salivary glands may result in xerostomia.

Q72. How do periapical radiographs help in diagnosis of systemic sclerosis ?
Ans. Extreme widening of the periodontal space around the roots of multiple or all teeth is associated with systemic sclerosis.

Q73. What are the other radiological findings of systemic sclerosis ?
Ans. In systemic sclerosis, unusual findings of resorption of angle of mandible and condyles of mandible is seen.

Q74. What are microscopic changes in periodontal ligament in systemic sclerosis ?
Ans. Microscopic features of periodontal ligament in systemic sclerosis include widening due to an increase of collagen and oxytalan fibers and hyalinization of collagen fibers. Number of connective tissue cells is reduced considerably.

Q75. What are the microscopic changes of skin in systemic sclerosis ?
Ans. Sclerosis of skin is characterized microscopically by thickening and hyalinization of collagen fibers, loss of

dermal appendages like sweat glands, atrophy of epidermis, and increased melanin pigmentation.

9.
VESICULOBULLOUS DISORDERS

Q1. What is Vesicle ?
Ans. Vesicle is lesion of mucosa or skin, and defined as well circumscribed, raised, fluid filled lesion measuring less than 5 mm in diameter.

Q2. What is bulla ?
Ans. Bulla is a well circumscribed, raised, fluid filled lesion measuring more than 5 mm in diameter.

Q3. What is pustule ?
Ans. Pustule is a lesion similar to vesicle orbulla but filled with purulent material.

Q4. What is the histological classification of vesicle ?
Ans. Histologically the vesicle can either be intraepithelial or subepithelial.
Intraepithelial vesicle is also known as suprabasillar type of vesicle. In intraepithelial vesicle the fluid is collected in prickle cell layer, whereas, fluid is collected below the basal cell layer in subepithelial vesicle.

Q5. Mention few diseases characterized by appearance of vesiles of bullae.
Ans. Vesiculo-bullous diseases include, Erythema multiform, pemhigus, Herpes virus infections, Herpes Zoster infections, Herpangina and bullous lichen planus.

Q6. Give an example of a disease in which subepithelial vesicles occur.
Ans. Bullous lichen planus, is a mucocutaneous disease in which bullae or vesicles are of subepithelial type. The antigen and antibody reactivity is located in basement membrane, causing degeneration of basal cell membrane.

Q7. **Give an example of disease in which the vesicles are intraepithelial type.**

Ans. Intraepithelial vesicles occur in Herpes virus stomatitis and pemphigus.

Q8. **Classify the vesiculo-bullous disease.**

Ans. Vesiculo-bullous diseases can be classified in many ways. In etiology based classification, the diseases can be grouped into –
  I.   Traumatic – Caused by burns
  II. Infections – Viral infections like herpes simplex, herpes zoster, herpangina, Hand foot mouth disease.
  III. Immunologic disorders like allergy, submucous fibrosis and lichen planus.
  IV. Developmental like Epidermolysis bullosa and psoriasis.
  V.   Miscellaneous diseases include the diseases with unknown or Multietiological factors like, erythema ultiform, pemphigus, benign mucous membrane pemphigoid and Steven-Johnson syndrome.

Q9. **What are the different herpes virus infections oral cavity ?**

Ans. There are six herpes viruses that cause infection in and around oral cavity. They are Herpes simplex virus (1 and 2 type), Varicella zoster, Cytomegalo virus, Epstein-barr virus, and human herpes virus-6.

Q10. **Which nucleic acid is present in herpes virus ?**

Ans. Herpes viruses contain a DNA nucleus and can remain latent in host cells.

Q11. **What is the composition of Herpes simplex virus ?**

Ans. The Herpes simplex virus is composed of four layers. They are an inner core of linear double stranded DNA, a protein capsid, the tegument, and lipid envelope containing lycoproteins that is derived from the nuclear membrane of host cells.

Q12. Which type of Herpes simplex virus causes oral cavity infections more often ?

Ans. Type 1 of Herpes simplex virus is responsible for infection of oral cavity.

Type-2 is mostly associated with infection of genitalia. However with changes is sexual behavior, the type-2 virus may rarely cause infection of oral cavity.

Q13. Write the clinical features of primary herpes simplex virus stomatitis.

Ans. Primary oral infection occurs in individuals with no prior infection with herpes simple virus, It occurs mostly in children between 6 months to 6 years. The incubation period is most commonly 5 to 7 days. Initial prodromal symptoms include pyrexia, acute gingivitis, headache and malaise. One or two days after prodromal symptoms, small vesicles appear on gingival, tongue and palate. The vesicles are small and fragile and rupture within few hours. Ruptured vesicles result in shallow ulcers. Segregated ulcers will appear as larger ulcerated area. Inflammation may be evident in pharyngeal area also. The nodes are enlarged, inflamed and tender.

Q14. What is the management of primary acute herpetic ginvivostomatitis ?

Ans. Scrapping from the base of vesicle are collected and placed on microscopic glass slide. This can be stained with giemsa, or papanicolaou stain and examined for multinucleated giant cells and ballooning degeneration of nucleus.

Q15. What is the management of primary acute herpetic gingivostomatitis ?

Ans. Acute perpetic gingivostomatitis causes severe pain and discomfort. Loss of fluid and difficult in taking liquids and normal fluids may lead to dehydration and the ulcerative lesions are prone for secondary infection. Acyclovir is the antiviral drug which may be useful in the managemtn of the acute lesions. Topical anaesthetics are used to reduce the pain. Antipyretic can be given to control pyrexia.

Q16. What is Recurrent herpes Labialis or stomatitis ?
Ans. Recurrent herpes Labialis is secondary or recurrent infection caused by activation of herpes simplex virus which remain latent in nerve roots or ganglion.

Q17. Write clinical features of recurrent herpetic stomatitis or labialis.
Ans. Recurrent herpes stomatitis or labialis is caused by activation of dormant virus by precipitating factors. These factors, include lowered resistance, fever, use of certain drugs, trauma, exposure to sun rays. The vesicles appear on oral mucosa and exposed part of upper lip. Labial lesions are more common than intraoral vesicles. They are few in number.

Q18. What is cold sore ?
Ans. Cold sore is a name given to vesicles or ulcers occurring recurrent herpes labialis. These lesions occur after the onset of fever.

Q19. What are lipschutz bodies ?
Ans. Lipschutz bodies are eosinophilic, ovoid, homogeneous structures within the nucleus. Thesea re seen in the cells collected from vesicles of herpetic gingivostomatitis.

Q20. Name the diseases caused by varicella zoster virus ?
Ans. Varicella Zoster virus causes two forms of disease. The primary infection causes chickenpox and secondary infection herpes zoster (shingles). In general chickenpox is a generalized form.

Q21. Write the clinical features of chickenpox.
Ans. Chickenpox is an acute viral disease. The incubation period is approximately two weeks. It usually occurs in children. The disease is characterized by prodromal symptoms of headache, anorexia, malaise and pyrexia. It is then

followed by maculopapular or vesicular eruptions of the skin. The eruptionusually begin on the trunk and spread to involve face and extremities. Vesicles rupture, form superficial crust and heal by desquamation.

Q22. Write the oral manifestations of chickenpox.
Ans. Intraoral mucosal lesions are not very common. Occasionally vesicles may appear on buccal mucosa, tongue, ingiva and pharynx. The vesicles are surrounded by erythema. The vesicles rupture forming small ulcers.

Q23. What is shingles ?
Ans. Herpes zoster or shingles is an acute viral infection caused by reactivation of herpes zoster virus. The virus remains latent in the nerve root ganglia.

Q24. Write the clinical features of Herpes Zoster infection.
Ans. Herpes zoster is an acute disease of extremely painful and incapacitating disease characterized by inflammation of dorsal root ganglia or extramedulary cranial nerve ganglia and associated with vesicular eruption of the skin or mucosa innervated by affected nerve. The disease mostly affects adults. Initally patients exhibit fever and malaise. Pain in the areas innervated by the nerve, precedes the appearance of vesicles. The vesicles do not usually cross the midline and are unilateral. Healin occurs after rupture of vesicles. Sometimes secondary infection may occur.

Q25. What are the oral manifestations of the herpes zoster infection ?
Ans. Herpes Zoster may involve the trigeminal nerve as well as sensory component of facial nerve. Vesicular eruptions occur on skin of the face or oral mucosa innervated by the affected nerve. The vesicles on oral mucosa rupture resulting ion erosive lesions. These lesion are unilateral and do not cross midline. The ulcers are painful and heal in 7 to 10 days.

Q26. What is Ramsay Hunt's Syndrome ?
Ans. Ramsay Hunt's syndrome is a form of herpes zoster infection of the geniculate ganglion. The virus remains latent in the ganglion. Reactivation of the irus, causes abnormalities related to sensory component of facial nerve. The clinical features include facial paralysis, pain and vesicular eruptions on external auditory meatus and pinna. Intraoral sites of pain and vesicular eruptions include oral mucosa of oropharynx.

Q27. What is the etiology of hand, foot and mouth disease ?
Ans. Hand, foot and mouth disease is caused by coxsackie virus.

Q28. Write the clinical features of Hand, foot and mouth disease.
Ans. Hand, foot and mouth disease is an acute viral diseas, mostly occurring in children. It is characterized by the appearance of maculopapular and vesicular lesions of the skin of feet, legs, arms and buttocks. The patients may also suffer from fever, lymphadenopathy, nausea and vomiting.

Q29. What are the oral manifestations of Hand, foot and mouth disease ?
Ans. Oral mucosal lesions are common occurrence in Hand, foot and mouth disease. Stomatitis is initial and common finding. It is followed by multiple vesicular eruptions which bread to form small, multiple ulcer. These may appear on oral mucosa of any area including gingival, hard palate, tongue and buccal mucosa.

Q30. What is Erythema Multiform ?
Ans. Erythema multiform is an acute form of dermatitis of unknown etiology and manifesting it self in different forms.

Q31. What is the etiology of Erythema Multiform /
Ans. There is no definite proved etiology which is responsible for protean manifestations. A variety of different agents

are known to precipitate an attack of the disease in number of individuals and it may appear spontaneously in others. The precipitating factors which may trigger the attack include drugs (like barbiturates, phenylbutazone and sulfonamides), vaccinations, radiation, fungal, bacterial and viral disease. The viral infections include herpes simplex virus infection.

Q32. What is target lesion ?
Ans. A concentric ring like appearance of the lesions, resulting form the varying shades of erythema occur on the skin in erythema multiform. These lesions are described as "Target" or "Iris" or "Bull's Eye" due to peculiar appearance.

Q33. Write the clinical features of Erythema multiform ?
Ans. Erythema multiform is an acute condition, with sudden onset of vesiculobullous eruptions. It may occur in different forms. It occurs chiefly in young adults, even though it may occur in any age. It affects males more often than females. The disease is characterized by appearance of macular, popular, vesicular or bullous eruptions commonly over the hand, arms, feet, legs, face and neck. These lesions on skin present a typical appearance of concentric rings whick are termed as target, iris or bull's eye lesion. Vesiculo-bullous lesions also occur in oral mucosa but these do not present as target appearance. The vesicles or bullae rupture leaving erosive or ulcerative lesions.

Q.34. What are the oral mucosal lesion of erythema multiform ?
Ans. In erythema multiform, oral mucosa is involved alongwith dermal lesions. In few cases however, the oral lesions may precede skin lesions. The disease may present in the form of erythematous macules, papules, vesicles or bullae.They may cause pain and discomfort. The vesicles and bullae rupture resulting in erosive or ulcerative lesions. These lesions bleed freely. The erosive lesions are covered with

coagulated crust. The lesions may appear on giniva, tongue, palate, lips and buccal mucosa.

Q35. What is Stevens Johnson syndrome ?
Ans. Stevens Johnson syndrome is a very severe bullous form of erythema multiform with wide spread involvement of skin, oral mucosa, eyes and genitalia.

Q36. What are the eye lesions in Steven-Johnson syndrome ?
Ans. Eye lesions include photophobia, conjunctivitis and corneal ulcerations.
Keratoconjunctivitis sicca also may occur.

Q37. What are oral mucosal lesions in Stevens Johnson syndrome ?
Ans. Oral mucosal lesions appear abruptly following occurrence of fever, malaise and skin eruption. Vesicles orbullae appear on oral mucosa which rupture and leave surfaces covered with a thick or yellowish exudates. These lesions are extremely severe, painful and cause difficulty in mastication. Ulcerations on lips may exhibit bloody crusting.

Q38. Mention the genital lesions Stevens Johnson syndrome ?
Ans. In Stevens Johnson syndrome the genital lesions include nonspecific urethritis, balanitis and in females vaginal ulcers.

Q39. What is Toxic epidermal necrolysis ?
Ans. Toxic epidermal necrolysis is an uncommon but serious, often fatal bullous drug eruption disease. It is so severe that large areas of skin peel off, giving the appearance of a wide spread scalding burn. Oral lesions appear similar to Stevens Johnson syndrome.

Q40. What is pemphigus ?
Ans. Pemphigus is a serious, and chronic mucocutaneous disease characterized by small vesicles orlarge bullae.

Q41. Mention the types of Pemphigus.
Ans. Several types of pemphigus have been reported. Four ofthese are well recognizd. These are pemphigus vulgaris, Pemphigus vegetans, pemphigus foliaceus and pemphilgus erythematosus.

Q42. What is the basic lesion of all the types of pemphigus ?
Ans. Vesicle or bulla is the basic lesion of all the types of pemphigus.

Q43. Which type of pemphigus usually exhibits oral mucosal lesion ?
Ans. Oral mucosal lesions mostly occur in pemphigus vulgaris and sometimes in pemphigus vegetans.

Q44. Describe the clinical features of pemphigus Vulgaris.
Ans. Pemphigus mostly occurs in age group of over 30 years. The incidence is equal in both the sexes. Pemphigus Vulgaris is characterized buy rapid appearance of bullae which enlarge by lateral spread. Initially lesion mayoccur on skin, over the trunk, arms and neck. Sometimes oral lesions may precede the skin lesions. The bullae which contain thin fluid may rupture leaving raw eroded areas. The characteristic feture is the positive NIKOLSKY'S sign. Nikolsky's sign is appearance of vesicle or bulla on lateral application of pressure over the skin or mucosa. Wider involvement may prove fatal due to loss of fluid and secondary infection. Sometimes it may show recovery and remission in few weeks.

Q45. Write the clinical features of pemphigus Vegetans.
Ans. Pemphigus Vegetans is considered as a variant of pemphigus vulgaris. The bullae rupture and the eroded area exhibit "Vegetations" These are covered by purulent exudates.

Q46. Write the clinical features of pemphigus foliaceus.
Ans. The oral manifestations in the type of pemphigus are uncommon. The skin lesions characterized by bullous lesions which rapidly rupture and dry leaving flakes and scales.

Q47. Describe the clinical features of pemphigus erythematosus.
Ans. Pemphigus vulgaris is a vesiculo-bullous disease, which is characterized by thin walled bullae, which rupture leaving eroded areas. These areas resemble seborrheic dermatitis or lupus erythematosus.

Q48. What type of bulla is seen in pemphigus ?
Ans. Pemphigus is characterized by bullae, which are intraepithelial. The fluid is collected within the epithelium above basal cell layer. These bullae are described as suprabasillar bullae or vesicles.

Q49. What are the Tzanck cells ?
Ans. Tzanck cells are acantholytic or degenerative cells which are found in vesicles or bullae in pemphigus. These cells are characterized by degenerative changes which include swelling and hyperchromatism of the nuclei. There is an increase in RNA in the cytoplasm. The acantholytic cells are produced by prevesicular edema and dissolution of intercellular attachments.

Q50. What is Tzanck test ?
Ans. Tzanck test is process of collection of acantholytic cells from vesicles or bullae and examination under microscope.

Q51. Describe the microscopic features of pemphitgus.
Ans. Initially pemphigus is charcterised by prevesicular edema and loss of intercellular bridges. Subsequently separation or split of epithelial cells from basal cell layer is seen. The vesicles and bullae are suprabasillar or intraepithelial. Fluid from bullae contains Tzanck cells, polymorphonuclear leukocytes nad lymphocytes. Pemphigus is characterized

by absence of inflammatory cell infiltration in connective tissue.

Q52. Write the findings immunofluorescent tests in pemphigus.
Ans. Direct immunofluorescent test is used to demonstrate the presence of immunoglobulins in the intercellular spaces or intercellular substance in the epithelium of the lesion or normal epithelium adjacent ot the lesion.
These immunoglobulins are IgG, IgA or IgM.

Q53. Write the management of pemphigus.
Ans. Management of pemphigus includes topical and systemic administration of corticosteroids. Antibiotics are used to control secondary infection.

Q54. What is Benign Mucous membrane Pemphigoid ?
Ans. Benign mucous membrane pemphigoid is a vesiculobullous disease of unknown etiology affecting oral mucosa and eye. It is also known as cicatricial pemphigoid or ocular pemphigus.

Q55. Describe the clinical features of cicatricial pemphigoid ?
Ans. The cicatricial pemphigoid occurs in older age group individuals. It affects females more often than males. Vesiculobullous lesions occur on oral mucosa and conjunctiva. These heal by scar formation. Mucous membrane of nose, larynx, pharynx, esophagus, vagina and penis may also be affected on few occasions. These are uncommon site. The most significant is development of adhesions between palpebral and bulbar conjunctivae.

Q56. What is the type of bulla in cicatricial pemphigoid ?
Ans. The bullae and vesicles are subepithelial type in cicatricial pemphigoid or benign mucous membrane pemphigoid.

Q57. Write the microscopic findings of lesions of cicatricial pemphigoid.

Ans. The microscopical features are nonspecific. There is no acantholysis. The separation or degeneration occurs at basement membrane below the epithelium. Therefore the vesicles or bullae are sub-epithelial and thick walled. Connective tissue exhibits inflammatory cell infiltration.

Q58. What is the location of antibodies in the lesion of cicatricial pemphigoid ?

Ans. Immunofluorescence studies have shown the presence of tissue bound basement membrane antibodies. Therefore they are seen along with basement membrane.

Q59. What is the differential diagnosis of cicatricial pemphigoid ?

Ans. The various conditions to be considered in dirrefential diagnosis of cicatricial pemphigoid include erythema multiform, bulluous lichen plnus, pemphigus vulgaris and bullous pemphigoid.

Q60. What are the drugs useful in the treatment of benign mucous membrane pemphigoid ?

Ans. Topical or systemiccorticosteroids are useful in the treatment o benin mucous membrane pemphigoid.

Q61. What is parapemphigus ?

Ans. Parapemphigus or bullous pemphigoid is another vesiculo bullous disease, considered to be variant of dermatitis herpetiformis.

Q62. Write the clinical features of parapemphigus ?

Ans. Parapemphigus or bullous pemphigoid is basically a disease of old age group. The skin lesions appear as generalized rash on limbs. It is pruritic. The rash may reamin for few weeks before appearance of vesicles and bullae. The vesicles and bullae are thick walled and also occur on abdomen, neck and legs.

Q63. What are the oral manifestations of parapemphigus?

Ans. The oral mucosal lesions in parapemphigous are not very common like either in pemphigus vulgaris or cicatricial pemphigoid. The lesion may be vesicles, bullae or erosive erythematous area. These may be present on gingival, buccal mucosa or other area of oral mucosa.

Q64. What is the type of bulla in parapemphigus ?

Ans. The vesicles or bullae are of sub-epithelial type in parapemphigus. Separation occurs at the junction of epithelium and basement membrane.

Q65. What is epidoermolysis bullosa ?

Ans. Epidemolysis bullosa is an uncommon dermatological disease in which vesiculo-bullous lesion develop spontaneously after a minor trauma. There are different forms of the disease.

Q66. Classify Epidermolysis bullosa.

Ans. Epidermolysis bullosa is classified into different forms. They are epidemolysis bullosa simplex, epidermolysis bullosa dystrophic, junctional epidermolysis bullosa, and epidermolysis bullosa acquisita.

Q67. Which of the types of epidermolyiss bullosa exhibit oral manifestation ?

Ans. Not all the types of epidermolysis bullosa are known to exhibit the oral manifestations. The oral mucosal lesions are more common in epidermolysys bullosa dystrophic.

Q68. What are the oral mucosal lesions of epidermolysis bullosa dystrophic ?

Ans. Bullae occur on the oral mucosa. These bullae are preceded by the appearance of white spots or erythematous areas. The bullae may be initiated by simple. Mild injuries or pressure or with even minor dental operative procedure. The bullae rupture leaving ulcers or erosisions which are painful. Scare formation may result in obliteration of sulci and restriction of movements of tongue.

10.

FACIAL PAIN AND NERVE DISORDERS

Q1. What is pain ?
Ans. Pain is an unpleasant sensory experience. It is a symptom.

Q2. What are the components of pain ?
Ans. Pain has two main components. One is organic and another is psycholofic.

Q3. Define pain.
Ans. The pain is unpleasant sensory and emotional experience associated with actual or potential tissue damage.

Q4. What is alodynia ?
Ans. Alodynia is pain due to a stimulus that does not normally produce pain.

Q5. What is Hyperalgesia ?
Ans. Hyperalgesia is an increased response to a stimulus that is usually painful.

Q6. What is Hyperaesthesia ?
Ans. Hyperaesthesia is an increased sensitivity to stimulation and does not imly a painful sensation but rather an augmented response to a specific sensory mode. (E.g. Tough, temperature and vibration).

Q7. What is causalgia ?
Ans. Causalgia is burning pain after traumatic injury to the nerve.

Q8. What is neuritic pain ?
Ans. Neuritic pain is pain occurring locally due to inflammation of nerves or nerve endings.

Q9. What is neuralgia ?
Ans. Neuralgia is pain occurring in tissues along the distribution of nerve.

Q10. What is paraesthesia ?
Ans. Paraesthesia is an abnormal or altered sensation (e.g. tingling).

Q11. What is Formication ?
Ans. Formication is a form of sensation or feeling of worms creeping below the skin.

Q12. What are the tests for assessment of pain ?
Ans. Pain is subjective experience Hence measurement of pain is not possible objectively. Even thouh pain cannot be measured irectly, various methods have been advocated that allow patients to communicate the amount of pain. These are useful is patient's care and evaluation. The methods advocated include (a) Visual analog scale (b) Category scale (c) Numeric Scale (d) McGill pain questionnaire.

Q13. What is visual analog scale ?
Ans. Visual analog scale is simple method of rating of pain. It consists of drawing a line of 10 cms markings. One end of line is marked as "No pain" and another is marked as most severe pain. The patient is asked to indicate the magnitude of pain on the scale. This can be used as a reference to compare the pain in future visits.

Q14. What is category scale ?
Ans. Category scale is simple grading of apin into four categories "None, mild, moderate and severe". The patient is asked to record the magnitude of pin in these categories.

Q15. What is numeric rating scale ?
Ans. In numeric rating scale, the magnitude of pain is graded or indicated by numbers.

Q16. What is McGill pain Questionnaires ?
Ans. McGill pain questionnaire (MPQ) is questionnaire where in the pain adjectives are arragned in 20 groups. The assessment is arrived from the markings by the patients.

Q17. Classify facial pain ?
Ans. Facial pain can be classified broadly into three groups,
1. Pain arising form diseases of orofacial structures.
2. Pain arising from disorders of nerves and central nervous system.
3. Pain arising in distant organs and referred to facial region.

Q18. Describe pain from hypersensitive dentine.
Ans. Dentine may be exposed due to various causes includein caries, inadequate filling, filling with marginal leakage and recurrent caries, fracture of tooth, abrasion, erosion and attrition. The pain is described as severe and sharp of shorter duration and always precipitated by contact of hot, cold or sweet food or beverages. Diagnosis is often easy as the cause can be diagnosed by either clinical or radiological examination.

Q19. Describe pain from acute pulpitis.
Ans. Acute pulpitis pain is severe, radiating pain with sudden onset or may be precipitated by hot or cold stimuli and lasts for longer duration. Patient usually recognizes as it is originating from tooth, but which often cannot be localized to a particular tooth. The pain is exacerbated by lying down position. Tooth is sensitive and responses early to electric pulp testing.

Q20. Describe the clinical features of giant cell arteritis.
Ans. Giant cell arteritis is of unknown etiology. IT can affect cranial arteries and temporal artery. Affected vessel show destruction of inner layer and middle layer may show

granulomatous inflammation and giant cells. The lumen may become blocked. Pulsations may be absent.

The disease affects mostly older age group and may be characterized by fever, malaise, pain in the temporal, occipital and scalp. Muscle pain may be present due ischemia. Muscles of mastication may be involved causing pain and difficulty in mastication.

Q21. What is MPDS ?
Ans.   MPDS is myofascial pain dysfunction syndrome. It is a disorder characterized by facial pain due to involvement of muscels of mastication. It simulates the clinical features of diseases of temperomandibular joint.

Q22. Write the etiology of MPDS.
Ans.   Etiology of myofascial pain dysfunction (MPDS) include spasm of muscles of mastication. Most often lateral pterygoid muscles and masseter muscle are involved. The spasm may result from either due to overcontraction or due to overwork leading to fatigue. Bruxism may be one of the findings. Depression, anxiety, stress emotional disturbances may be precipitating factors in muscle disorders.

Q23. Describe the clinical features of MPDS.
Ans.   MPDS is characterized by pain in preauricular, temporal and occipital region. In addition limitation of jaw opening, deviation of midline and clincking sound in TMJ are common findings. In addition to these poritive findings, there are certain negative findings which equally important in the diagnosis of MPDS. These are absence of organic changes and radiological changes in temperomandibular joint.

Q24. Write the management of MPDS.
Ans.   The management of MPD necessarily include treatment of both emotional and physical components of the disorder. As the stress or emotional disturbances are predisposing or underlying causative factors, the emphasis shall be laid on identifying and relieving these factors. Local anaesthetic

spray can be used for anaesthetizing the affected muscle and thereby allowing the patient to stretch the muscle or muscles. Application of ice for 10 minutes and stretching the muscles 3 to 4 times a day may help. Nonsteroidal anti inflammatory drugs maybe presceibed. A mind tranquilizers or sedatives may be useful. Appliances like bite guard or occlusal splints may be used to correct parafunctional habits. Transcutaneous electric nerve stimulation (TENS) has also been advocated in certain cases of MPDS.

Q25. Which are the neuralgia occurring in orofacial region ?

Ans. The most common among the neuralgias of orofacial region is trigeminal neuralgia. Other neuralgias include glossopharyngeal neuralgia, geniculate ganglion neuralgia and post herpetic neuralgia.

Q26. Describe the clinical features of trigeminal neuralgia.

Ans. Idiopathic trigeminal neuralgia or tic douloureux has been recognized as an extremely painful disorder of trigeminal nerve. It mostly involve mandibular and maxillary branches. Pain occurs in the region of innervation of branch of the nerve. Recurrent episodes of severe, lancinating, shock like unilateral pain of very short duration for few seconds occur. Even though the pain is of a very short duration, the patient may present history of long duration, due to post pain phase of fear psychosis. The episode of pain may be precipitated by non-noxious stimulation of certain areas by normal function or activity. These areas are called trigger zones. The act of speech, washing face, shaving or brushing may precipitate the painful episode. After each episode there is a refractive pain free period. This ma range from few hours, few days to few months. Trigeminal neuralgia occurs more frequently in women and right side. The painful episodes may range from several per day to any few per year. Typically the painful episode do not occur in night during sleep.

Q27. What is Trigger Zone ?
Ans. Trigger zone is an area in the course of its distribution, stimulation of which precipitates the attack of pain in neuralgias. Trigger zones are located on the surface of either skin or muscle.

Q28. Write the medical treatment of trigeminal neuralgia.
Ans. Treatment of idiopathic trigeminal neuralgia can be medical or surgical. Medical treatment shall precede the surgical intervention. Medical treatment include use of carbamezapine in the dose of 100 mg to 200 mg per day to a maximum dose of 1200 mg per day. The treatment should commence with smaller dose and should gradually increased every 48 hours till optimum level of maintaining prolonged pain free period. After few days of treatment the dose may be reduced gradually to a level of maintenance dose.

Q29. What are the other forms of treatment of trigeminal neuralgia ?
Ans. Injection of absolute alcohol around the nerve and into the ganglion and peripheral neurectomy are also useful forms of treatment.

Q30. What are the other drugs found effective in idiopathic trigeminal neuralgia ?
Ans. Other than carbamezapine, beclofen in the dose of 50 mg to 80 mg per day in divided doses in found to be effective. This can be used in combination with carbamezapine.

Q31. What are the side effects of carbamezapine ?
Ans. Initially the drug may cause drowsiness and vertigo. The drug is cytotoxic. Long use of carbamezapine may cause aplastic anemia and leucopenia. Hence periodic hematologic examination is required during the treatment.

Q32. What are the types of Glossopharyngeal neuralgia ?
Ans. Depending upon the area involved the glossopharyngeal neuralgia may be either otic type or pharyngeal type.

Q33. Describe the clinical features of Glossopharyngeal neuralgia.
Ans. Glossopharyneal neuralgia is less common and less severe than trigeminal neuralgia. The localtion of trigger zone and pain follows the distribution of IX cranial or glossopharyngeal nerve. The location includes pharynx, posterior area of tongue, ear, infrauricular area. The pain is triggered by chewing and sallowing.

Q34. What is the differential diagnosis of Glossorpharyngeal neuralgia ?
Ans. Trigeminal neuralgia, geniculate neuralgia and Eagle's syndrome may simulate certain common features and shall be considered in differential diagnosis.

Q35. What is Geniculate Neuralgia ?
Ans. Geniculate neuralgis is painful episodes occurring in the areas innervated by sensory component of facial nerve. The pain occurs in the ear, pinna and less frequently soft palate. It is uncommon neuralgia.

Q36. Name the syndrome associated with Geniculate neuralgia.
Ans. Herpes zoster viral infection involving the Geniculate ganglion results in facial nerve palsy and vesicles on pinna, internal auditory canal and soft palate. This is referred as ramsay Hunt syndrome.

Q37. What is post herpetic neuralgia ?
Ans. Unlike other neuralgia which are mostly characterized by recurrent painful episodes of shorter duration, the post herpetic neuralgia is a persistent pain that conti nues even after healing of herpes zoster eruptions. The pain of severe lancinating and burning occurs over the innervated area of involved nerve. It is unilateral in distribution. There are no trigger zones.

Q38. What is treatment of post herpetic neuralgia ?
Ans. In post herpetic neuralgias, short term, high dose corticosteroid therapy and tricyclic antidepressant therapy have be found useful.

Q39. What is atypical facial pain ?
Ans. Atypical facial pain is poorly localized and atypical to distribution of sensory nerve.

Q40. What is the etiology of atypical facial pain ?
Ans. Etiology of atypical facial pain is not known, It may represent an important aspect of depression or psychological abnormality. The patients with atypical facial pain may exhibit different forms of depression like endogenous depression, atypical depression, anxety neurosis, obsessional neurosis or hysteria.

Q41. What is endogenous depression ?
Ans. Endogenous depression is a form of depression wherein individual wakes up early, unable to sleep and loss appetite. Such paietnes may be self critical, which may even proceed to delusion of punishment.

Q42. What is atypical depression ?
Ans. It is a form of endogenous depression wherein additional features of irritability, lethargy, and fatigue dominate over other features.

Q43. What is anxiety neurosis ?
Ans. These patients are aware of psychological tension building within and such tension may precipitate a wide spectrum of unfounded physical symptoms. This is more often seen before an important event in a person's life.

Q44. What is obsessional neurosis ?
Ans. The individuals with obsessional neurosis are always preoccupied by thoughts sufferings. Here the feelings and thoughts cannot be removed from mind. The feelings of

suffering are usually exaggerated at higher proportion than real symptoms. Such patients usually enumerate history n chronological organic features may be mild or absent.

Q45. Describe Hysteria.
Ans. In hysteria the individual's symptoms may be initiated and potentiated for the gain which he or she may obtain from them. Such patients usually have a doting relative or friend who perhaps in more concerned about the suffering than patient himself.

Q46. Describe the clinical features of atypical facial pain.
Ans. Patients suffering from atypical facial pain exhibit the symptoms of depression. The nature and location of pain may vary from time to time and usually unrelated to organic disease. The pain is atypical to distribution and course of sensory nerves. The pain may be dull to severe and of long duration.

Q47. What is differential diagnosis of atypical facial pain?
Ans. The differential diagnosis of atypical facial pain include periodic migranious neuralgia, myofacial pain dysfunction syndrome, sphenopalatine neuralgia, maxillary sinusitis, retrobulbar neuritis and cranial arteritis.

Q48. What is the etiology of periodic migrainous neuralgia ?
Ans. Exact etiology of this conditions is unknown. It is of vascular origin characterized by vascular constriction and then dialation, due to biochemical changes. Exact nature of biochemical changes are not known.

Q49. Write the clinical features of periodic migrainous neuralgia ?
Ans. Unlike miratinous pains which is more common in woman, the periodic migrainous neuralgia occurs more frequently in men. The pain strats suddenly and is of severe in nature. It may start around eyes, temporal region, extending to face. Nausea is common but vomiting does

not occur. The attacks of painful episodes generally occur once in 24 hours, more often in night waking up the patient. Hence it is also referred to "Alarm clock" headache.

Q50. What are the associated phenomena of periodic miranous neuralgia ?
Ans. There are number of associated phenomena which may occur along with facial pain in periodic migrainous neuralgia. The affected area or side feels hot an may even exhibit sweating. Epiphora and sensation of nasal block with rhinorrhea may occur. There may even be photophobia.

Q51. What is the treatment of periodic migrainous neuralgia ?
Ans. Various durgs have been used in the management of periodic migrainous neuralgia. Ergotamine preparations containsing ergotamine 1-2 mg and caffeine 100 m is common found effective. Transquillizer and sedative like diazepam 2 to 5 mg dose and antihistamine like chlorpheniramine maleate 5 mg are also used in the management of periodic migrainous neuralgia.

Q52. Mention few syndromes related with facial pain.
Ans. Myofascial pain dysfunction syndrome, Eagle's syndrome and trotter's syndrome.

Q53. What is Eagle's syndrome ?
Ans. Eagle's syndrome or stylalgia is characterized by pain while swallowing. This is caused either due to elongation of styloid process or due t classification of stylomandibular or stylohyoid ligaments.

Q54. What is Trotter's syndrome ?
Ans. Trotter's syndrome is characterized by facial pain in the middle third of face caused by invovlemetn of maxillary nerve due to carcinoma of nasopharynx.

Q55. Classify the disorders of facial nerve or seventh cranial nerve.

Ans. The disorder of facial nerve can be divided into:
1. Paralysis (a) upper motor neuron lesions (b) Lower motor neuron lesion.
2. Sensory branch disorders – (a) Ramsay Hunt Syndrome and (b) Post herpetic neuralgia.
3. Special senses: Taste sensations.
4. Miscellaneous – Frey's syndrome.

Q56. What is the etiology of upper motor neurone lesions of facial nerve.

Ans. Cranial tumors, hematoma and injuries of brain causing damage to cerebropontic tract or upper motor fibers of supranuclear fibres of facial nerve may cause upper motor neurone diseases.

Q57. What is the lower motor neuron disorder of facial nerve?

Ans. The diseases which affect the facial nerve below the level of nucleus in pons are considered as lower motor neuron lesions. Pontic lesions, Disseminated sclerosis, hematoma, tumors, compression of facial nerve in the facial canal, tumors of parotid gland, injury to peripheral branches, Herpes zoster of geniculate ganglion, and sarcoidosis of parotid gland cause the facial nerve paralysis.

Q58. Name the syndrome associated with sarcoidosis of parotid gland?

Ans. Heerfordt's syndrome is associated with sarcoidosis of parotid glnd and facial nerve palsy.

Q59. Write the differences between upper motor neurone lesions and lower motor neurone lesions of facial nerve.

Ans. *Upper Motor Neurone Lesions* (a) Lesions are located in C.N.S. above the nucleus of the facial nerve in the pons. (b) Ther are involvement of more than one nerve and hence resultant signs and symptoms involve many organs. (c) Effects are seen on contralateral side. (d) Of the facial muscles, the muscles of lower two-thirds of face are involved; as the muscles of foreheads are innervated from nerve fibers of both the sides. (e) Lacrimation and taste may not be effected.

Lower Motor Neurone Leisons (a) Lesions are located below the nucleus and along the course of the nerve. (b) Mostly affects facial nerve and sometimes sixthe cranial nerve also is involved. (c) Effects are seen on the same side. (d) Whole one side of face affected as nerve fibres from both the sides travel in one and same nerve. (e) Taste and lacrimation may be affected depending on the location of injury along the course of the nerve.

Q60. What is Hyperacusis ?
Ans. Hyperacusis is increased or exaggerated hearing. It may be caused by paralysis of the stapedius muscle.

Q61. What is Schirmer's test ?
Ans. Schirmer test is used to test the lacrimation. A-3 mm wide strip of litmus paper is placed in the lower conjunctival fornix. In normal lacrmation, about 15 mm of litmus paper gets wet in one minute.

Q62. Does the emotional expression in the face affected in facial nerve palsy ?
Ans. Emotional expression in the face may be affected in frontal or temporal regions are also involved in the lesions associated with upper motor nuclear pathway or supranuclear pathway of facial nerve. Emotional expression is not affected in facial nerve paralysis of lower motor neuron lesions.

Q63. Write the clinical findings of facial nerve involvement of lower motor neuron type.
Ans. Muscles of face on one side of the face show loss of function (paralysis). Even though frontal region muscles have bilateral supply they are also paralysedas there is ony one common path in lower motor neurone. The other features include reduced lacrimation and hyperacusis. These findings are not always present/ Depending on the

location and level of lesions these findings may be present. If the lesion is below the pontic level to above geniculate ganglion, lacrimation may also be affected along with loss of taste and hyperacusis. The level of involvement below the geniculate ganglion, spares the lacrimal flow. If the lesion is below the chorda tympani, even the taste is not affected. The lesion below the stapedium nerve, the hearing is also not affected.

Q64. What is Bell's palsy ?
Ans. Bell's palsy is common type of facial nerve paralysis of lower motor neurone type. It is named after Sir Charles Bell, the early nineteenth century anatomist.

Q65. Write the clinical features of Bell's palsy.
Ans. Bell's palsy occurs equally in both the sexes and may occur at any age. It mostly affects on side but alos may occur bilaterally. Onset may be sudden and most patients associate the onset with exposure to cold wind. In majority of cases all the muscles on affected side exhibit paralysis. Patients are unable to close the eyes, wrinkle the forehead, close the mouth and blow the whistle. Attempt to close the eyes results in rolling up of eye ball exposing white part, which is known as "Bell's Sigh". Muscles of the face on affected side are dragged to normal side. Saliva continues to dribble from the angle of the mouth on affected side. While eating, food collects in the vestibule on affected side. Lacrimation, taste may be affected depending on the location of defect.

Q66. Describe the management of Bell's Palsy.
Ans. In acute cases anti-inflammatory drugs including short-term corticosteroids are used. Preventive measures shall be taken to avoid eye infection by bathing eye frequently. Temporary tarsorrhaphy may be needed to support the muscles. Massaging of muscles is advocated. To prevent disuse atrophy the electric nerve stimulation is advocated. Surgical decompression of nerve may be done in certain cases where compression of facial nerve occurs.

Q67. What is Glossodynia ?
Ans. Glossodynia is a term used to indicate pain in the tongue.

Q68. What is Glossopyrosis ?
Ans. Glossopyrosis is a term used to indicate burning sensation on tongue.

Q69. What is stomatopyrosis ?
Ans. Stomatopyrosis is burning sensation of oral mucosa. It is also referred to as burning mouth syndrome.

Q70. What is Ageusia ?
Ans. Ageusia is complete loss of taste perception.

Q71. What is Dysgeusia ?
Ans. Dysgeusia is a used to indicate altered or distorted taste sensation.

Q72. What is Cacogeusia ?
Ans. Cacogeusia is a bad taste.

Q73. What is the etiology of Dsgeusia ?
Ans. There are number of etiological factors which alter the taste. These may be grouped as local and systemic. Local factors include loss of papillae due to thermal, chemical and mechanical injuries.
Other local factors include fungus infection, poor oral hygiene, use of complete dentures and orthodontic applicances. The systemic factors include blood disorders like anemia, in which taste buds get atrophic, central nerve disorders, Cranial nerve disorders, metabolic disorders and psychological disorders.

Q74. What are the etiological factors for burning mouth syndrome ?
Ans. The burning mouth syndrome may be caused by variety of local and systemic causes. Some of these may cause observable local tissue changes where as some do not show any organic changes. Local abnormalities include thermal and chemical injuries, allergies to food and

denture, local irritating factors, poor oral hygiene, cnadidal infection, oral submucous fibrosis, Lichen planus, erythroplakia, atrophic changes in oral mucosa, metabolic disorders, and hormonal disorders. Blood disorders like anemia ma cause atrophic changes on oral and lingual mucosa leading to burning sensation. Local tongue lesions like geographic tongue, scrotal or fissured tongue may also be responsible for burning sensation of tongue. In idiopathic burning mouth and neuralgic disorders local tissue changes may not be present.

Q75. What is Frey's Syndrome ?
Ans. Frey's syndrome is an unusual phenomenon which arises as a result of damage to the auriculo-temporal nerve and subsequent re-inneration of sweat glands by parasympathetic salivary fibers. This is also referred as Auriculo-temporal syndrome or Gustatory sweating disease.

Q76. What is the etiology of Frey's syndrome ?
Ans. The abnormality may follow surgical intervention of parotid gland or mandible which may result in damage to Auriculo-temporal nerve. During the regeneration of the damaged nerve, parasympathetic salivary nerve supply develops innerating sweating glands. This is an uncommon disorder.

Q77. Write the clinical features of Frey's syndrome.
Ans. The patients usually exhibit flushing and sweating on temporal region on affected side during eating. The sweating becomes more severe due to spicy foods. The sweating is characterized by its unilateral character on affected side. Parental administration of pilocarine results is severe sweating and sweating is absent when atropine is administered.

Q78. What are the causes of atrophy of muscles ?
Ans. The various causes which may likely to cause atrophy of muscles include disuse, ageing, cachexia, denervation, nutritional disturbances, metabolic disorders and muscular dystrophies and hypotonias.

Q79. What is Muscular Hypertrophy ?
Ans. Muscular hypertrophy refers to the increase in size of the muscle due to an increase in size of muscular fibers. The increase in size of the muscle may also occur due to increase in interstitial connective tissue. This is referred to as pseudohypertrophy.

Q80. What are the causes of muscular hypertrophy ?
Ans. The muscular hypertrophy may occur due to developmental defects, functional disturbances, inflammation, infections, metabolicdisturbances and neoplasia.

11.

CYSTS OF ORAL CAVITY

Q1. Define a cyst ?
Ans. Cyst is a pathological cavity having epithelial lining wall and containing fluid or semisolid material

Q2. What is pseudocyst ?
Ans. Pseudocyst is pathological cavity containing fluid or semisolid material but lacking epithelial lining.

Q3. Classify the cysts of orofacial structures.
Ans. Cysts of orofacial structures may be classified in different ways depending on etiological process, tissue of origin or location.

Q4. Classify cysts depending on location.
Ans. Cysts may occur either in jaw bones or surrounding soft tissues.

Q5. Classify the cysts depending on etiology.
Ans. Depending on etiology, the cysts of orofacial structures are broadly classified as developmental and inflammatory.

Q6. Classify the cysts based on tissue of origin.
Ans. Cysts are classified broadly as odontogenic and non-odontogenic based on wheather originating from tooth forming or other tissue respectively.

Q7. Mention few cysts occurring in soft of orofacial region.
Ans. Thyroglossal duct cyst, dermoid cysts, branchial cysts, Bohns nodules and Epstein pearls are few examples of soft tissue cysts.

Q8. Classify the cysts occurring in jaw bones.
Ans. In jaw bones the cysts can be classified into two groups 1. odontoenic 2. Non-odontogenic.

Q9. Name odontologenic cysts of jaw bones.
Ans. Primordial cysts, dentigerous cysts, radicular cysts, and odontogenic keratocysts are few odontogenic cysts.

Q10. What are the fissural cysts of jaw bones ?
Ans. Fissural cysts are those occurring from the epithelial remnants at junctions of various processes. These occur from the entrapped epithelial cells and appear in locations of union of various processes. These are known as fissural or inclusion cysts. These are developmental in origin.

Q11. Name the few fissural cysts.
Ans. The fissural cysts include mid palatine cysts, globulomaxillary cysts and mid-mandibular cyst.

Q12. What are the non-odontogenic cysts ?
Ans. Cysts which do not arise from the tooth tissue but arise from epithelial cells entrapped in various locations. These include fissural cysts.

Q13. Name the cysts associated with missing teeth.
Ans. Primordial cysts and odontogenic keratocysts occur from enamel organ before commencement of formation of hard tissues, hence the tooth fails to form. Cysts originate from enamel organ. However dentigerous cysts develops after the tooth has formed. Hence it is associated with impacted but clinically missing tooth.

Q14. What are the odontogenic cysts ?
Ans. The odontogenic cysts are those cysts, which are derived from the epithelium associated with the development of dental apparatus (Tooth).

Q15. What is the source of epithelium for development of odontogenic cysts ?
Ans. Epithelium from following sources may be involved in development of odontogenic cysts.
1. Tooth germ, 2. Reduced enamel epithelium of crown, 3. Cells rests of malassez and 4. Remnants of dental lamina.

Q16. What is the acceptable basis of classification of odontogenic cysts ?
Ans. Type of odontogenic cysts depends on the stage of development of tooth, at which cyst develops. Hence acceptable basis of classification of odontogenic cysts is stages of odontogenesis during which they originate.

Q17. Classify the odontogenic cysts of oral cavity.
Ans. The following classification of odontogenic cysts fulfills most of the criteria.
1. Primordial cyst
2. Dentigerous cyst
    (a) Eruption cyst
3. Periodontal cyst
    (a) Apical (b) Lateral periodontal cyst
    (c) Residual cyst
4. Gingival cyst
    (a) Cysts of new born (Epstein pearls, Bohns nodule)
    (b) Cyst of adults
5. Odontogenic Keratocysts
6. Calcifying odontogenic cyst

Q18. What are the odontoenic cysts which are developmental in origin ?
Ans. Odontogenic developmental cysts include primordial cysts, odontogenic keratocyst, gingival cysts of infants, gingival cysts of adults, dentigerious cyst, eruption cyst and calcifying odontogenic cyst.

Q19. what are the odontogenic cysts of inflammatory in origin ?
Ans. Inflammatory odontogenic cysts include Radicular cysts (apical and lateral), residual cysts, and paradental cyst (uncommon)

Q20. What are the gingival cysts of infants ?
Ans. Gingival cysts of infants are small cysts occurring during infancy. They are multiple and nodular like structures found on alvelolar ridge mucosa and palatal mucosa. They are derived from remnants of dental lamina.

Q21. Name the gingival cysts of infants.
Ans. Epstein's pearl are small cysts arising during embryogenesis as a consequence of entrapment of epithelial residues along the midline of palate. They appear as small multiple white nodular structures.

Q22. What are the Epstein's pearls ?
Ans. Epstein's pearls are small cysts arising during embryoenesis as a conswquence of entrapment of epithelial residues along the midline of palate. They appear as small multiple white nodular structures.

Q23. What are the Bohn's nodules ?
Ans. Tiny, multiple cysts of palate in infants were described by Bohn in 1866. These are believed to occur from epithelial remnants of minor salivary glands on palate. Therefore they are seen on posterolateral halves of palate.

Q24. What are the locations of dental lamina cysts of infants ?
Ans. The dental lamina cysts develop from remnants of dental lamina hence are located on alveolar ridge.

Q25. What is the pathogenesis of primordial cyst ?
Ans. Primordial cyst develops through cystic degeneration and liquefaction of the stellate reticulum in an enamel organ beforeformation of enamel and dentine. Therefore

primordial cyst occurs in place of a tooth either of normal complement or supernumerary tooth.

Q26. In which area, the primordial cyst occurs most often ?

Ans. Common location for the primordial cyst to occur is mandibular posterior region. It may occur from enamel organ of mandibular third molar.

Q27. Write clinical features of primordial cyst.

Ans. Primordial cysts occurs in young adults. It is most often asymptomatic unless it is secondarily infected or grows to large size causing expansion of bone. The tooth is found missing.

Q28. Describe the radiographic features of primordial cyst.

Ans. In radiographs, the primordial cyst appears as a round or ovoid well demarcated radiolucent area. The radiolcent area may exhibit sclerotic border. The radiolucent design is unilocular most often however it may also be multilocular. The lesion is seen in place of missing tooth.

Q29. Write the microscopic appearance of primordial cyst.

Ans. Microscopically, the primordial cyst presents as cystic cavity surrounded by epithelial lining and wall of collagen fibers. The epithelial lining may be nonkeratinised and may exhibit prominent spinous layer with elongeated retepegs. In some instances, the epithelium may present with a layer of orthoor parakeratin.

Q30. Write the treatment of primordial cyst.

Ans. Surgical removal of the cyst and curettage of bone is the treatment of choice in primordial cyst.

Q31. What is distinctive feature of odontogenic keratocyst ?

Ans. Exceedingly high rate of recurrence is very distinctive feature observed in odontoenic keratocyst.

Q32. Write clinical features of odontoenic keratocyst.
Ans. Odontogenic keratocyst occurs in young adults. The mandible is invariably affected more often than maxilla. Posterior part is common site. There are no typical clinical features. However pain and paraesthesia are associated with swelling. Expansion of mandible may not be prominent feature as the cyst spreads in anteroposterior direction rather than laterally.

Q33. Describe the radiological appearance of odontogenic keratocyst.
Ans. Odontogenic keratocyst may appear as either a unilocular or multilocular radiolucent area surrounded by sclerotic border. This border may be smooth or scalloped. The radiolucent lesion may be large, and may cover a wider area.

Q34. Describe the microscopic features of wall of odontoenic keratocyst.
Ans. Wall of odontogenic keratocyst is thin. The lining epithelium is made up of 6-10 cell ayers, and exhibits parakeratinisation of surface, which is corrugated. The basal cells are prominent and are palisaded. This is characteristically described as having "picket fence" or "tombstone" appearance.
Surrounding connective tissue wall often shows small islands of epithelium similar to that of cystic wall. Thse epithelial islands may form daughter cysts and are responsible for high recurrence rate of odontogenic keratocyst.

Q35. What are contents of odontoenic keratocyst ?
Ans. Lumen of the keratocyst may be filled with a thin straw colored fluid or with a thicker creamy material representing keratin.

Q36. What is the treatemtn of odontogenic keratocyst ?
Ans. Treatment of odontogenic keratocyst include complete removal cyst with its wall and curettage of bone.

Q37. How does the presence of multiple odontogenic keratocysts, make it essential to evaluate the patients medically ?

Ans. Multiple odontogenic keratocysts are associated with Jaw cyst-Basal cell nevus-Bifid rib syndrome.

Q38. What is Jaw cyst-Basal cell nevus-Bifid rib syndrome ?

Ans. Jaw cyst-Basal cell nevus-Bifid rib syndrome is a complex syndrome which includes a great variety of abnormalities. It is also known as basal cell nevus syndrome, Gorlin-Goltz syndrome.

Q39. Write clinical feature of Jaw cyst-Basal cell nevus-Bifid rib syndrome.

Ans. The abnormalities in jay cyst basal cell nevus-Bifid rib syndrome may include variety of changes involving multiple systems. The bony and dental anomalies include presence of multiple odontogenic keratocysts, mandibular prognathism and bifid ribs. The cutaneous anomalies include basal cell carcinoma, palmar and plantar keratosis and dermal calcinosis. The ophthalmologic anomalies include hypertelorism, congenital blindness and internal strabismus. The neurologic abnormalities include mental retardation, dural calcification, and congenital hydrocephalus. The sexual abnormalities include hypogonadism in males and ovarian tumors in females.

Q40. What are the types of radicular cyst ?

Ans. Radicular cysts are associated with roots of teeth. They can be either periapical (associated with apex of tooth) or lateral periodontal cyst (associated with lateral surface of the root). Radicular cysts may remain in the bone itself after removal of tooth, sch cysts are known as residual cysts.

Q41. What is the prerequisite for the periapical cyst ?

Ans. Necrotic pulp is the prerequisite for the periapical cyst. Hence such cyst is always associated with non vital tooth. Howewver if the cyst is associated with necrotic pulp of one root in multirooted teeth, such teeth still may give positive response to vitality tests.

Q42. What is the source of epithelial lining in radicular cyst ?

Ans. Epithelial lining of radicular cysts originate from the cell rests of malassez which are remnants of root sheath of Hertwig On rare occasions, it is possible that the source of epithelium may differ. It may derive from maxillary sinus lining (respiratory epithelium) if periapical lesion is close to sinus, oral epithelium if the cyst is associated with fistulous tract or it may derive from oral epithelium proliferating apically from periodontal pocket. However these are rare possibilities.

Q43. Write clinical features of periapical cyst.

Ans. The periapical cysts are common. They are mostly associated with maxillary anterior teeth which are mor prone for traumatic injuries, resulting in necrosis of pulp. The cysts are asymptomatic unless large in size or secondarily infected. The large cyst may cause external swelling. Infected cyst may cause sign and symptoms of inflammatory lesion. Invariably the associated tooth is found to be nonvital.

Q44. What is the pathogenesis of periapical cyst.

Ans. Periapical cyst is located at the apex of root with necrotic pulp. Cyst develops from the periapical granloma. The initial reaction leading to cyst formation is a proliferation of cell rests of Malassez. As this proliferation continues, the mass of epithelial cells become separated further and further from their source of nutrition and as a result of this undergo degeneration or necrosis and liquefy forming cyst.

Q45. Write the radiographic features of periapical cyst.

Ans. Radiologically periapical cyst appears as well circumscribed radiolucent area measuring more than one centimeter in diameter and located at the apex. Radiolucency may exhibit the cortication indicating slow progress. Lamina dura is continuous with the border of the lesion. Lamina dura around the apex is absent.

Q46. Mention the microscopic appearance of wall of periapical cyst.
Ans. Epithelial lining of periapical cyst is made up of stratified squamous type. Thickeness may vary from few layers of cells to thick. Ther is no keratin formation. Hyaline bodies or Rushton bodies may be found in epithelium. Connective tissue that forms the wall is made up of parallel bundles of collagen fibers.

Q47. What are the Rushton bodies ?
Ans. Rushton bodies or Hyalin bodies are found in epithelium of periodontal cysts. These are tiny linear shaped bodies which appear amorhous in structure, eosinophillic in reaction and are brittle in nature. These are found to be morphologically and histologically similar to erythrocytes. Therefore it is suggested that they arise from thrombus formation in small capillaries being formed from these erythrocystes.

Q48. What is the incidence of lateral periodontal cyst ?
Ans. Lateral periodontal cyst is uncommon condition, but well recognized separate cystic entity.

Q49. Which is the common site of lateral periodontal cyst?
Ans. Lateral periodontal cyst most often occurs in mandibular premolar region.

Q50. Describe the pathoenicity of lateral periodontal cyst (lateral radicular cyst).
Ans. Lateral periodontal cysts appear to arise from lateral surface of erupted tooth. The possibilities of mechanism of development of this cyst include origin from proliferation of cell rests of Malassez in periodontal ligament, origin as a primordial cyst from supernumerary enable organ, origin initially a dentigerous cyst developing on lateral surface of the crown and as tooth erupts it assumes position on

lateral surface of tongue, and finally it may originate from the proliferation cells remants of dental lamina which are in port functional state.

Definite stimulus for the proliferation of cell rests of Malassez of periodontal ligament and remnants of dental lamina is not known.

Q51. Write clinical features of lateral periodontal cyst.
Ans. Lateral periodontal cyst usually occurs in adults. There is predilection for occurrence in males over females. It invariably occurs in mandibular premolar region. It may also occur in maxillary incisor areas. The majority of cases do not show nayclinical signs and symptoms. It becomes symptomatic either after it growns into a larger size orafter it gets infected. Large cyst may cause divergence of roots and convergence of crowns and expansion of cortical plates. The associated tooth invariably is vital.

Q52. Describe the radiological features of lateral periodontal cyst.
Ans. Lateral periodontal cyst appears in radiographs, as well demarcated circular or oval radiolucency, situated on the lateral surface of roots. The radiolucency may exhibit sclerotic border. The roots on either side may be pushed apart.

Q53. Write the microscopic features of lateral periodontal cyst.
Ans. Microscopic features of lateral periodontal cyst are essentially a cavity lined by epithelial lining, surrounded by connective tissue wall. Epithelial lining may be made up of single flate cells to several cells of stratified squamous type. Many of the lining cells exhibit clear, vaculolated, glycogen rich cytoplasm. Focal thickening of lining due to proliferation of cells may be observed. Connective tissue wall is made up of bundles of collagen fibers. Rests of dental lamina are sometimes found in the connective tissue wall.

Q54. How does the primordial cyst differs from dentigerous cyst ?
Ans. Primordial cyst originates from enamel organ before formation of hard tissues whereas dentigerious cyst originates after completion of crown.

Q55. Mention few common features of primordial and dentigerous cysts.
Ans. Both the cysts originate during formation of tooth. In both the cysts, concerned tooth is found to be missing clinically. Both the cysts are found mostly in young adults.

Q56. What is the pathogenesis of Dentigerios cyst ?
Ans. Dentigerous cyst originates from accumulation of fluid between reduced enamel epithelium and surface of crown of tooth. Thus it forms after completion of crown formation. Rarely dentigerous cyst may originate by proliferation and cystic transformation of islands of epithelium in connective tissue wall of dental follicle.

Q57. Write clinical features of dentigerous cyst.
Ans. Dentigerious cyst is more common than primordial cyst. It mostly occurs in young adults. The most common sites for this cyst to occur are mandibular third molar, maxillary third molar and maxillary canine areas. Tooth involved is found missing clinically. Initially the cyst is mostly asymptomatic. Epansion of boen becomes evident as cyst grows in size. Secondarily infected cyst may exhibit signs and symptoms of pain and swelling. The diagnosis of dentigerous. Cyst is mostly found from routine radiographs cyst is associated with impacted and unerupted tooth. This may also be associated with odontoma.

Q58. Describe radiological features of dentigerous cyst ?
Ans. In radiographs, the dentigerious cyst appears radiolucent area round the crown of impacted or unerupted tooth. The radiolucent area is well demarcated and exhibits radiopaque broder. The cyst may eb larger, pushing or displacing the tooth involved. The cystic cavity may be so large as to involve ramus as well. If the cyst is in relation

to odontoma, the radiolucency may surround either mass of radiopacity (complex odontoma) or multiple tiny radiopaque small teeth like structures (compound odontomal), Radiolucency may rarely exhibit multilocular appearance.

Q59. Write microscopic features of dentigerous cyst.
Ans. There is no characteristic microscopic appearance. Cystic lining is made up of thin layer of stratified squamous epithelium. Rete pegs generally are absent, except in cases that are secondarily infected. The connective tissue wall is thick and is made up of very loose fibrous connective tissue or sparsely collagenised myxomatous tissue. Mucous secreting cells may be found occasionally.

Q60. What are the potential complications of dentigerous cyst?
Ans. Development of ameloblastoma and carcinoma are the potential complications likely to occur from dentigerious cyst. Development of muco-epidermoid carcinoma was also reported on few ocsions. This could be from mucous secreting cells found in epithelial lining of dentigerous cyst.

12.

PRE MALIGNANT CONDITIONS AND LESIONS

Q1. What is a pre malignant lesions ?
Ans. Pre malignant lesion is defined as a "Morphologically altered tissue in which malignancy is more likely to occur than in its apparently normal counterpart. Leukoplakia and erythroplakia are two pre malignant lesions of oral mucosa.

Q2. What is pre malignant condition ?
Ans. Pre malignant condition is defined as "a generalized state associated with a significantly increased risk of malignancy". Oral submucous fibrosis and sideropenic dysphatgia are the two pre malignant conditions.

Q3. What are the changes seen in epithelial dysplasia ?
Ans. Changes seen in epithelial dysplasia include loss of polarity of basal cells, increased nuclear cytoplasmic ratio, droplet shaped rtepeges, increase in mitotic firuges, the presence of mitotic figures even in superficial layers, nuclear hyperchromatism, cellular pleomorphism, keratinisation of individual cells or groups of cells and loss of cohesion between cells.

Q4. What is carcinoma in situ ?
Ans. Carcinoma in situ represents a precancerous dyskeratotic changes within the epithelium of skin or oral mucosa. It is also called intraepithelial carcinoma.

Q5. Write the clinical features of carcinoma in situ.
Ans. Clinically carcinoma in situ may resemble leukoplakia, erythroplakia or ulcerated lesion. These may occur on floor of mouth, tongue, lips and buccal mucosa. It is more common in males than in females.

Q6. Write the microscopic features of carcinomain situ.
Ans. Carcinoma in situ or intraepithelial carcinoma is characterized by a remarkable range of avriation in histologic appearance. Dysplastic changes in epithelium include increased mitotic figures in all the layers, increased nuclear cytoplasmic ratio, hyperchromatic nucleus, basal cell hyperplasia, hyperkeratosis and individual cell keratinisation.

Q7. What is Leukoplakia ?
Ans. Leukoplakia is a nonscrapable white lesion of oral mucosa measuring more than 5 mm and which cannot be characterized clinically and histologically as any other entity. It is mostly tobacco related.

Q8. What is the etiology of leukoplakia ?
Ans. Tobacco consumption is the main cause of the leukoplakia. However other causes like irritation from sharp margin tooth, consumption of spices and spirits, bad oral sepsis, vitamin deficiency, endocranial disturbances, syphilis and actinic radiation have been implicated.

Q9. Write clinical features of leukoplakia.
Ans. The leukoplakia of oral mucosa shows considerable variation in size, location and clinical appearance. It is more common in men and older age group. However it may be seen in younger age group. These nonscrapable white patches exhibit predilection to certain sites like buccal mucosa, and commissures but may also occur on alveolar mucosa, tongue, lips, palate, floor of mouth and gingival. Leukoplakia is described as having three main clinical forms. They are homogemeous, nodular and verrucous.

Q10. What is homogeneous leukoplakia ?
Ans. Homogeneous is a clinical form of leukoplakia which presents as relatively consistent uniform pattern. Sometimes the surface may be described as corrugated, wrinkled or papillomatous.

Q11. What is nodular leukplakia ?
Ans. Nodular leukoplakia refers to a mixed red and white lesion in which small keratotic nodules are scattered over an atrophic mucosa. It is also referred to as granular, speckled or non homogeneous. This variety has higher changes of transformation to malignancy.

Q12. What is verrucous leukoplakia ?
Ans. Verrucous leukplakia is a term used to describe oral mucosal white lesion charcterised by multiple papillary projections on the surface. It is nonscrapable. Extensive lesions of verrucous carcinoma are sometimes referred to as florid oral papillomatosis.

Q13. Leukoplakia is a premalignant lesion. Leukoplakia of which site have more potential to turn into malignancy ?
Ans. The leukoplakia of floor of the mouth, lips and tongue are known to transform more often into mkalignancy.

Q14. Write the microscopic features which help in diagnosis of leukoplakia.
Ans. Diagnosis of leukoplakia is made when adequate clinical and histological examination fails to provide evidence for an alternative diagnosis. How ever important microscopic features of leukpplakia is cellular dysplasia. The dysplastic changes include hyperkeratosis or hyperparakeratosis. Cellular pleomorphism cellular atypia, drop shaped retepeges, hyperplasia of basal cell layer, increase nuclear cytoplasmic ratio and hyperchromatosis.

Q15. Write the management of leukoplakia.
Ans. Initial step in th management of leukplakia is identifying local irritating or causative factors and systemic factors.

These local factors shall be eliminated and systemic factors shall be corrected. Small lesion shall be removed surgically. For many years systemic administration of vitamin A or its synthetic analogues like retinoic acid, have been advocated as an adjunctive treatment for an extensive leukoplakia lesion.

Q16. What are the toxic effects of retinoic acid ?
Ans. Toxic effects of retinoic acid includes facial erythema, dryness and peeling off of the skin and conjunctivitis.

Q17. How does retinoic acid help in leukoplakia ?
Ans. Retenoic acid or vitamin A are known to have diverse biologic effects among which immunoenhancement, promotion of epithelial differentiation, and antioxidant activity have been suggested as mechanism underlying the effectiveness of retinoids in the treatment of leukoplakia.

Q18. What is erythroplakia ?
Ans. Erythroplakia is any area of reddened, velvety textured mucosa that cannot be identified on the basis of clinical and histologic examination as being caused by inflammation or any other disease process.

Q19. Mainly are the different modes of use of tobacco ?
Ans. Mainly tobacco is used either in the form of smokeing or nonsmoking tobacco. Smoking tobacco is used in the form of cigarettes, cigar, pipe smoking, Chutta, beedi, hukka and reverse smoking. Smokeless tobacco is used in the form of chewing tobacco holding of "pinch" (finely ground tobacco), or wad (coarsely cut tobacco) in buccal or labial vestibule, and nass (snuff) used for local application as well as for inhaling. The chewing tobacco is used either with or without Pan and Khaini. Mixture of pan and tobacco are held in buccal vestibule. Chewing tobacco is also available in the form of *Pan Masala or Ghutka.*

Q20. What is Lichen planus ?
Ans. Linchen planus is a relatively common mucocutaneous disease, which may exhibit manifestation either on skin or oral mucosa or on both together.

Q21. Describe the skin lesions seen in lichen planus ?
Ans. The skin lesions of lichen planus are mostly constant and are flat violaceous papules with fine thin scales on the surface. These lesions cause itching sensation.

Q22. What is the etiology of lichen planus ?
Ans. Definite etiology of lichen planus is not known. It is most often present in individuals suffering from stress. Etiology also involves cell medicated, immunologic reaction.

Q23. What are the types of lichen planus ?
Ans. Clinically lichen planus is described in different forms. Hypertrophic, bullous, atrophic, erosive and reticular.

Q24. Mention the common sites of skin lesions in lichen planus ?
Ans. This skin lesions may occur on any part of skin, however the most common site being flesor surfaces of forearms and wrists, inner aspect of knees and thighs and sacral area of trunk. They are bilaterally symmetrical.

Q25. What types of mucosal lesions are seen in lechen planus ?
Ans. Maculopapular erosive lesions are seen in lichen planus.

Q26. Describe the clinical appearance of reticular form of lichen planus.
Ans. The reticular form of lichen planus consists of slightly elevated, fine papules, arranged in lace like lines. The linear arrangement may appear as radiating lines or annular (ring like). These fine radiating lines are referred to as striae of wickham. Reticular form is the commonest form among all the types of lichen planus. The lesions may be seen on buccal mucosa, tongue and alveolar mucosa and present bilaterally.

Q27. Describe the clinical features of atrophic lichen planus.
Ans. Atrophic forms of lichen planus occurs with less frequency. Clinically it appears as smooth, red, poorly defined areas with peripheral striae. It may be asymptomatic or have burning sensation. Alveolar mucosa, buccal mucosa may be effected.

Q28. What is the location of antigen antibody reaction in lichen planus ?
Ans. Immunofluorescent tests have demonstrated localization of antibody at basement membrane.

Q29. What are the civatte bodies ?
Ans. Civatte bodies are degenerated epithelial cells of phagocytosed epithelial cell remnants within the macrophage. These appear as round eosinophillic globules. Civatte bodies are also known as clolloid bodies, hyaline bodies or fibrillar bodies.

Q30. Describe the microscopic features of lichen planus.
Ans. Lichen planus exhibits typical microscopic features. These include hyperparakeratosis or hyperorthokeratosis, thickening of granular layer and acanthosis. Intracellular edema of spinous layer may be present sometimes. Retepegs develop saw tooth appearance. The basal cell layer may show liquefaction degeneration resulting in appearance of thin band of eosinophillic coagulum. Civatte bodies are present in epithelium. Subepithelial layer may show infiltration of inflammatory cells in papillary zone of lamina propria. These inflammatory cells are arranged in band like arrangement.

Q31. Write the management of lichen planus.
Ans. Various forms of management including medications, surgery and cryotherapy have been advocated. Most often the lesion in lichen planus are diffused, hence surgery and cryotherapy may not be accessible. Medical treatment includes antihistamines, cortisones and retinoids. These

could be mostly used locally either in the form of cream, gel, aerosol spray, or solution. Reticular form may show regression on its own to reappear again. However erosive form most often requires active medication.

Q32. What is the oral submucous fibrosis ?
Ans. Oral submucous fibrosis is a chronic condition characterized by fibrosis in subepithelial zone (Juxta epithelial layer).

Q33. What is the etiology of oral submucous fibrosis ?
Ans. Use of chillies and arecanut have been thought to play a role in etiology of oral submucous fibrosis. Underlying nutritional deficiency enhances the chances of occurrence of oral submucous fibrosis. Active ingredient of chillies "capsaicin" has been associated with submucous fibrosis. However many workers found no correlation between the sue of chillies and occurrence of oral sumucous fibrosis. Arecanut chewing is predominantly associated with causation of oral submucous fibrosis. Arecoline is an active principle of arecanut. Arecanut is used with or without combination of pan, catechu, tobacco and lime. Immunologic abnormality has also been suggested as one of the etiological factor in oral submucous fibrosis. Many investigators suggested that the patients with oral submucous fibrosis have a genetic predisposition, which renders their oral mucosa susceptible to chronic inflammatory changes and fibrosis if they chew arecanut.

Q34. Write the clinical features of oral submucous fibrosis.
Ans. Oral submucous fibrosis affects elderly age group. However younger age group using arecanut also have been reported suffering from oral submucous fibrosis. It affects people of Asian origin. It can caffect any part of the oral cavity. It most often affects buccal mucosa, retromolar areas, soft palate, lips and tongue. It results in restriction of movements. The onset is slow, with burning sensation and intolerance to spicy food. Later vesicle formation and erythematous areas may develop. Subsequently the

mucosa appears pale or blanched. Gradual stiffening of the oral mucosa results in few years with formationj of fibrotic bands. The fibrosis may extend all over the oral cavity resulting in restricted movements of tongue as well as difficulty in opening the mouth. Oral mucosa exhibits marble like appearance and leathery texture.

Q35. Write the microscopic features of oral submucous fibrosis.
Ans. Oral submucous fibrosis shows characteristic microscopic features sonsisting of atrophic epithelium and juxtaepithelial hyalinization and fibrosis. The epithelium may exhibit keratinisation. The rete pegs are absent in atrophic epithelium. In advanced cases it may appear as ribbon like stirp. Atrophic epithelium may show dysplasia.

Q36. What is the management of oral submucous firbosis?
Ans. Various medical and surgical form of Management have been advocated with variable rate of success. Intralesional injection of corticosteroids, fibrinolysin, and hyaluronidase have been advocated. Systemic administration of corticosteroids and vitamin "A" have been advocated. Surgical management include cutting of fibrotic bands.

Q37. What is Plummer-Vinson syndrome ?
Ans. Plummer-Vinson syndrome is a form of iron deficiency anemia, occurring in elderly women.

Q38. When was the Plummer-Vinson syndrome first described ?
Ans. Severe form of iron deficiency anemia characterized by dysphagia was first describe by Plummer is 1914 and later by Vinson in 1922 under the term "Hysterical dysphagia".

Q39. Write the oral manifestation of Plummer Vinson syndrome.
Ans. Plummer-Vinson syndrome or sideropenic dysphagia is a severe form of iron deficiency anemia occurring in elderly women. It is characterized by signs and symptoms of

anemia, like fatigue, loss of weight, pallor, loss of appetite, koilonychias and oral manifestations The oral manifestations include loss of filiform papillae and fungiform papillae leading to bald tongue, stomatitis, atrophic oral mucosa, cracks and fissures at the corners of mouth and esophageal strictures causing dysphagia. Predisposition of this condition to the development of carcinoma is well established.

Q40. Write the laboratory findings of Plummer-Vinson syndrome.

Ans. Blood examination shows hypochromic microcytic anemia. Erythrocyte count may be normal or reduced marginally. Bone marrow examination may not show any megaloblasts which are typical to pernicious anemia. Serum iron is low. Achlorhydria is a common finding. The anemia of iron deficiency can be confirmed by lack of a reticulocyte response following administration of vitamin B12.

13.

TUMORS

Q1. Classify tumors of orofacial region.
Ans. Tumors of orofacial region are broadly classified as
1. Odontogenic
    a. epithelial in origin.
    b. connective tissue in origin.
    c. mixed.
2. Non-odontogenic
    a. epithelial in origin.
    b. connective tissue in origin.
Tumors of oral cavity can also be classified as benign or malignant base on bistopathological appearance, behaviour and prognosis.

Q2. Mention few example of odontogenic tumors of oral cavity.
Ans. Odontogenic tumors may originate either from epithelial tissue, or ocnenctive tissue or from both.
1. *Epithelial:* Enameloma, Ameloblastoma
2. *Connective tissue:* Dentinoma, cementoma, cementoblastoma, cementifying fibroma.
3. *Mixed:* Odontoma, Ameloblastic Fibroma

Q3. Name non-odontogenic tumors of oral cavity.
Ans. a. *Epithelial in origin:* Papilloma, Adenoma, Carcinoma.
b. *Mesenchymal in origin:* Fibroma, Lipoma, Fibrosarcoma, Neurofibroma, Osteoma, Chondroma, Haemangioma, Lymphangioma, Adenocarcinoma, Melanoma.

Q4. Name few benign Neoplasia of oral cavity.
Ans. Ameloblastoma, Clacifying epithelial odontogenic tumor, Adenomatoid ameloblastoma, Dentinoma, Odontomas,

Cementoma, Odontogenic fibroma, Papilloma, Pleomorphic adenoma, Fibroma, Lipoma, Neurofibroma. Neurilemmoma, Leiomyoma, Osteoma, Chondroma, Haemangioma and Lymphanigioma.

Q5. Name few examples of malignant tumors of oral cavity.

Ans. Carcinoma, Fibrosarcoma, Osteosarcoma, Primary intraosseous carcinoma, Chondrosarcoma, Adenocarcinoma, Pleomorphic adenoma, Metastatic carcinoma.

Q6. What is hamartoma ?

Ans. Hamartoma is an abnormal proliferation of tissues of structures native to the part.

Q7. Give examples of hamartoma of orofacial region.

Ans. Odontoma, haemangioma and lymphangioma are few examples of hamartomas occurring in orofacial region.

Q8. What is enameloma ?

Ans. In true sense enameloma is not a tumor but is referred to tumor in literature due to the fact that it constitutes a small and focal growth of enamel. It is also referred as enamel pearl. It appears as tiny globule of enamel which is found near bifurcation or trifurcation roots. This enamel nodule sometimes contains core of dentine and pulp.

Q9. What is ameloblastoma ?

Ans. Ameloblastoma is true neoplasm derived from enamel organ. It is described by Robinson as a tumor that is "usually unicentric, nonfunctional, intermittent in growth, anatomically bening and clinically persistent."

Q10. What is the other name of Ameloblastoma ?

Ans. Ther term "Ameloblastoma" was suggested by Churchill in 1934, to describe a tumor originating from enamel forming apparatus. Earlier this tumor was known as "Adamantinoma" as coined by Malassez in 1885. The term adamantinoma implies the formation of hard tissue and such tissue is not found in this tumor.

Q11. What is the pathoenesis of ameloblastoma ?
Ans. Exact nature of stimulus for formation of tumor is not known. The ameloblastoma is believed to origin from the (a) Cell rests of enamel organ, either remnats of the dental lamina or remnants of Hertwig's sheath (cell rests of malassez) (b) epithelium of dentigerous cyst (c) enamel organ (d) basal cells of oral epithelium or (e) heterotopic epithelium in other parts of the body (like pituitary body).

Q12. Describe clinical features of ameloblastoma.
Ans. Incidence of ameloblastoma is equal in both the sexes. It may occur in any age between 20 years and 40 years. Most of the cases in mandible than maxilla. Posterior part of mandible is the more common site. The typical ameloblastoma begins insidiously as a central lesion wihci rown slowly causing expansion of bone rather than destruction and perfeoration of cortical plates. The ameloblastoma rarely causes discomforting signs and symptoms; except for growth in size. Break down of oral mucosa does not occur even in very large lesions. Expansion of bone occur both on buccal and lingual surfaces of bone.

Q13. Describe the radiographic features of ameloblastoma.
Ans. Radiographic appearance of ameloblastoma is typically presents as multilocular radiolucent ares and described as honeycomb appearance. The periphery of the lesion is most often smooth. Thinning of cortical plates may be seen.

Rarely the ameloblastoma may present as unicystic radiolucency.

Q14. Describe the histologic appearance of ameloblastoma.

Ans. Microscopic appearance of ameloblastoma basically resembles enamel organ and different stages of histogenesis. A number of different types of microscopic appearances have been describe. They are follicular, plexiform, basal cell type, acanthomatous and granular cell types.

The follicular ameloblastoma is composed of many small discrete islands composed of a peripheral layer of cuboidal or columnar cells resembling ameloblasts. The layer of columnar cells enclosed a central mass of polyhedral, loosely arranged cells resembling the stellte reticulum. In few instrnces the stellate reticulum type mass may disinterate resulting in cystic formation. In the plexiform ameloblastoma, the ameloblast like tumor cells are arranged as network of interconnection stands of cells. Stellate reticulum like cells are arranged in between and are less prominent than in follicular type.

In the acanthomatous type, the polyhedral central cells undergo squamous metaplasia, sometimes with formation of keratin.

In the granular cell type, there is marked transformation of cytoplasm, usually of central polyhederal cells, so that it take coarse, granular and eosinophillic appearance. The granular appearance often extends to columnar cells as well these cytoplasmic granules represent aggregation of lysozymes. The basal cell type appear more like basal cell carcinoma of skin. The epithelial tumor cells are more primitive and less columnar and are arrangedgenerally in sheets.

The connective tissue stroma in all these type generally do not differ and is made of bundles of collagen fibres arranged loosely or densely.

Q15. Write the treatment of Ameloblastoma.

Ans. Complete removal of tumor is ideal form of treatment. IT could be accomplished by either radical or conservative excision. Radical excision is more often advocated.

Q16. What is the prognosis of Ameloblastoma ?
Ans. As metastasis is absent and it is locally invasive tumor, proper and complete removal of diseased tissue is possible. Hence it has good prognosis.

Q17. Which lesions are considered in differential diagnosis for radiographic appearance of Ameloblastoma ?
Ans. Odontogenic keratocyst, calcigying odontogenic cyst, calcifying epithelial odontogenic tumor, and adenomatoid ameloblastoma can be considered in differential diagnosis of radiographic appearance of ameloblastoma.

Q18. What is Pindborg tumor ?
Ans. The calcifying epithelial odontogenic tumor was first described as separate entity in 1956 by Pindborg. Therefore it is referred as Pindborg tumor.

Q19. Write clinical features of calcifying epithelial odontogenic tumor.
Ans. Calcifying epithelial odontogenic tumor (C.E.O.T.) most frequently occurs in middle age with not significant sex predilection. It is twice more common in mandible than maxilla and the prevalence in the molar region is three times than that of premolar region. The tumor initially does not cause any sign and symptoms therefore the patients are most often asymptomatc in initial stages and may present with painless swelling. In few cases the swelling is associated with clinically missing tooth.

Q20. Write the radiographic appearance of calcifying epithelial odontogenic tumor.
Ans. Calcifyin epithelial odontogenic tumor presents varying radiographic picture depending on the amount of calficiation. Lesion appears as well demarcated radiolucent area with foci of radiopacity. Irregular radiopaque shadows of trabeculae may traverse in many directions. Scattered flecks of calcifications throughout radiolucency have given rise to the descriptive term of a "driven snow". In some

instances the lesion is unilocular radiolucency with an impacted tooth and foci of calcification.

Q21. Decribe the microscopic picture of calcifying epithelial odontoenic tumor.

Ans. Calcfying epithelial odontogenic tumor is composed of polyhedral epithelial cells either packed closely or arranged in island of cells in fibrous connective tissue storma. The tumor cells show well defined cell border with a finely granular eosinophilic cytoplasm. Inter cellular bridges are often prominent. Another characteristic feature of the calcifying epithelial odontogenic tumor is the presence of calcification. The calcification. The calcification appwars to occur in some instances in globules of the amyloid like material.

Q22. What is the treatment of calcifying epithelial odontogenic tumor ?

Ans. Like in ameloblastoma, treatment of calcifying epithelial odontogenic tumor include complete removal of tumor. However radical resection may not necessary due to less invasive nature of tumor.

Q23. What is Adenomatoid odontogenic tumor ?

Ans. The Adenomatoid odntogenic tuor is benign odontogenic tumr characterized by the formation of ductlike structures by the epithelial component of tumor.

Q24. Write clinical features of Adenomatoid odontogenic tumor.

Ans. Adenomatoid odontogenic tumor occurs in young adults more often. It shows more predilection to female sex than males. Unlike C.E.O.T., this tumor is more common in maxilla than in mandible and occurs in anterior region than posterior region. Maxillary caine region is commnly involved. The tumor presents as swelling in the region of clinically missing tooth. In general the swelling is asymptomatic. It most often presents clinical features similar to dentigerous cyst.

Q25. Write the radiographic feature of Adenomatoid Ameloblastoma.

Ans. Adenomatoid ameloblastoma appears as unilocular radilucency similar to dentigerous cyst. Cystic wall appears to be attached on the root instead of cementoenamel junction. Hence ncreased length of the tooth appears to be in radiolucency. Scattered rediopaque foci are seen in the radiolucent area.

Q26. Write microscopic picture of adenomatoid ameloblastoma.

Ans. Adenomatoid ameloblastoma consist of polyhedral, or spindle or cuboidal shaped epithelial cells arranged in duct like or tubular arrangement. Droplets of unusual amorphous eosinophilic material are frequently found between the epithelian cells arranged in columns. Foci of calcification are often seen scattered throughout the tumor. Lesion is encapsulated.

Q27. What is dentinoma ?

Ans. Dentinoma is extremely rare and uncommon tumor. It originates from odontogenic tissue. There has been difference of opinion regarding the dentinoma being a true tumor.

Q28. Write radiographic features of dentinoma.

Ans. Radiographic features of dentinoma are not specific. The lesion may appear as radiolucent area exhibiting calficied solitary mass or multiple masses resembling odontoma.

Q29. Write clinical features of Ameloblastic fibroma.

Ans. Ameloblastic fibroma is believed to involve both epithelial and mesenchymal odontogenic tissue. It affects mostly younger individuals. Mandible is mostly involved than maxilla. Posterior region particularly premolar involved than anterior. The lesion is mostly asymptomatic except for casing sloly progressing expansion of the involved bone.

Q30. Write mocroscopic appearance of Ameloblastic fibroma.
Ans. Ameloblastic fibroma is seen microscopically to be composed of small and thin island of odontogenic epithelium dispersed randomly thgouhout mesodermal tissue that resembles dental papilla.

Q31. What are the odontomes ?
Ans. Odontomes are the malformations comprising a mass of the dental hard and soft tissues and which ar of limited growth, they are believed to be hamartomas.

Q32. Name few odontomes.
Ans. Complex odontome and compound odontome. Invaginated and evainated odontomes are also sometimes categorized as odontomes however, they are in true sense are abnormalities or malformations of teeth.

Q33. What is complex odontoma ?
Ans. Complex odontoma is malformation and collection of dental hard tissue and soft tissue as a mass. Ename, dentine and cementum are formd and arranged irregularly without any systematic arrangement.

Q34. What is compound odontoma ?
Ans. Compound odontoma is odontoma where in the malformations of dental tissues are arranged in the shape of tiny, multiple denticles. The denticles resemble small teeth. These denticles are arranged in fibrous capsule.

Q35. Write clinical features of odnotomas.
Ans. Odontomas are invariably asymptomatic and diagnosed from routine radiographs. These occur in younger individual. The odontomas are associated with unerupted and impacted teeth. Therefore cliincaly one can find a missing tooth. Odontomas sometimes may cause hard swelling. Mandibular last molar and maxillay conines are most common sites.

Q36. Write radiographic features of odontomas.
Ans. Complex odontoma appears as rapiopaque irregular mass of varying size surrounded by radiolucent zone, indicating encapsulation. This is associated with impacted and unerupted tooth.
Compound odontoma appears as a radio-opaque mass made up of multiple, tine tooth like structures at the crown of impacted and unerupted tooth. The radio opaque lesion exhibits clear radiolucent area surrounding it.

Q37. What is pathogeniesis of odontogenic myxoma ?
Ans. Odontogenic myxoma is bening tumor of jaw bones presumably originating from odontogenic mesenchymal tissue. It is an uncommon tumor.

Q38. Write clinical features of odontogenic myxoma.
Ans. Odontogeic myxoma is bening tumor, which grows slowly, it is invariably presents as painless swelling causing mild expansion of bone. Once the swelling becomes large, it may result in loosening and displacement of teeth. Youngh adults are most often affected. It occurs in mandible more than maxilla. It may sometimes be associated with missing or unerupted tooth.

Q39. Write the microscopic features of odontogenic myxoma.
Ans. Predominant component in odontoenic myxoma is loosely organized mucinous tissue in which the stellatic cells are usually relatively sparsely distributed. Strands and islands of odontogenic epithelium are randomly distributed throughout the lesion.

Q40. What are the cementomas ?
Ans. Cementomas are the group of pathological conditions related to cemental dysplasia. It is not always celar as to where line of demarcations should be dran between the cementum or cementum like tissue abnormalities and ture cementoma, the neoplasm.

Q41. Mention the condition which are grouped under cemental dysplasia or cementoma.

Ans. Benign cementoblastoma, periapical cemental dysplasia, cementifying fibroma and gigantiform cementoma are conditions grouped under cementoma.

Q42. What is benign cementoblastoma ?

Ans. Benign cementoblastoma is recognized as being a neoplasm of cemental tissue and therefore it is sometimes referred to as "true cementoma".

Q43. Write the clinical features of benign cementoblastoma.

Ans. Benign cementoblastoma occurs in younger age group. Roots of molars and premolar are the common sites. Associated tooth is vital unless co-incidentally involved. Benign cementoblastoma remains asymptomatic. Growth in size may cause expansion of bone. It is mostly detected on routine radiographs.

Q44. Write radiographic features of benign cementoblastoma.

Ans. The tumor appears as a well circumscribed dense radiopaque mass attached to the apex of root. The radio-opacity is surrounded by thin radiolucent rim. Lamina dura may be absent.

Q45. Write microscopic picture of benign cementoblastoma.

Ans. Benign cementoblastoma is made up of sheets of cementum like substance. It sometimes resembles cellular cementum and sometimes as a globular mass of giant cementicles. It may also contain variable amount of soft tissue component consisting of fibrillar, and vascular elements. Tumor is surrounded by layer of cementoblasts and occasionally by osteoclasts.

Q46. What is periapical cemental dysplasia ?

Ans. Periapical cemental dysplasia is a lesion rather common, and believed to origin either from the cementum or as a result of unusual reaction of periapical bone. It is not considered as a true neoplasm even though it is also referred as cementoma in literature.

Q47. What is the etiology of cementoma or periapical cemental dysplasia ?

Ans. Even though exact etiology is unknown, the contributory factors incude trauma, occlusal trauma, mild infection of tooth or hormonal imbalance.

Q48. Write clinical features of periapical cemental dysplasia.

Ans. Teeth involved wth periapical cemental dysplasia are invariably asymptomatic and vital unless otherwise co-incidentally involved. It may occur in younger individual and women are more affected than men. Mandibular incisor teeth are the commoner site than others. Mandibular premolar are also affected. Maxillary teeth are somehow not affected. Multiple teeth are affected together. These lesions are mostly diagnosed from routine radiographs.

Q49. Describe the pathological changes occurring in periapical cemental dysplasia.

Ans. The periapical cemental dysplasia shows wider tissue changes from its earlies stages which is known as osteolytic stage shows destruction of bone and fibrous tissue deposition around apices of teeth. In the second stae the fibrous tissue and connective tissue shows changes with commencement of calcification. There appears to be number of cementoblasts. This second stage is known as cementoblastic stage. The stimulus for the initiation of calcification is unknown.

The third stage which is known as matue stage is characterized by the deposition of increased aount of cemetum like tissue as a mass around apices of roots.

Q50. Describe the radiological featues of periapical cemental dysplasia.

Ans. The three stages of periapical cemntal dysplasia exhibit three different radiographic appearance.

During first stage (osteolytic stage) the lesion appears as radiolucent area at apices of teeth, resembling periapical granuloma or cyst. The radiolucent area is well demarcated.

During cementoblastic stage, the lesion exhibits certain foci of radio opacity scattered in radiolucency.

The mature stage of periapical cemental dysplasis, appears as well dermarcated radio-opaque mass at the apices of roots. The radio-opaque mass is surrounded by radiolucent zone.

Q51. Mention the lesion considered in differential dianosis of radiological appeace of matured cementoma.

Ans. Various lesion which present as radiopaque shadow in relation to roots are considered in differential diagnosis of matured cementoma. These are hypercementosis, chronic sclerosin osteomyelitis, and enostosis.

Q52. Write the clinical features of central cementifying fibroma.

Ans. Central cementifying fibroma may occur at any age but more common in younger age group. The aerage age group being 30 to 40 years. Increased predilection for female sx in noted. Mandible is more often involved than maxilla. The lesion presents no signs and symptoms till it grows larger in size to cause expansion of bone. Teeth may et displaced. Overlaying mucosa appears normal.

Q53. What is pathogenesis of cementifying fibroma ?

Ans. Central cementifying fibroma is neplasm of bone. There exists confusion as to weather cementifying fibroma and ossifying fibroma are one and the same or different. It has been suggested that both represent same entity with different tissue formations. It is either cementum or bone. The etiologic factor is unknown.

Q54. Descruve the microscopic features of cementfying fibroma.

Ans. Microscopic picture of cementifying fibroma shows presence of many delicate interlacing collagen fibers, interspersed by large numbers of active fibroblasts and cementoblasts. These cells may show mitotic activity but don not show much pleomaorphism. The lesion also shows presence of foci of cementum like tissue which appeas basophilic. These are irregularly round, elongated or oval in shape. Initially they are separate and later may coalesce forming wider areas of calcification. In few tumors, bone may be present instead of cementum.

Q55. How does cementifying fibroma appears in radiograph ?

Ans. Initial lesion which is mostly composed of fibrous tissue, appears as radiolucent area which is well demarcated and well circumscribed. As the lesion progresses with formation of cementum or bone, the radiolucent area exhibits foci of radiopacities. As the calcified tissue becomes coalesced into a large mass, the lesion may present as round or oval radiopawque mass within the radiolucency. Expansion of lower border of mandible may be seen, which is characteristic for diagnosis as the expansion is in confiratory to the outline of radiopaque mass.

Q56. Which are the commonest bening tumors of soft tissue in oral cavity ?

Ans. Among the tumors occurring in oral cavity, the fbroma and papilloma are the most common benign tumors arising from soft tissue elements.

Q57. Write the clinical features of Fibroma.

Ans. Fibroma is tumor of connective tissue origin and common benign tumor. It appears as elevated, nodular lesion of normal color. It is sessible and sometimes may be pedenculated. Surface appears smooth. Fibroma is slow growing and usually is symptomatic. The consistency is either firm or soft. It occurs on gingival, buccal mucosa, tongue and lips.

Q58. Describe the microscopic picture of fibroma.
Ans. Histologic appearance of Fibroma exhibits bundles of interlacing collagenous fibers interspersed with varying number of fibroblasts, fibrocytes and small blood vessels. Surface of the fibroma is covered by a layer of strafified squamous epithelium, which shows flattening of retepegs. On few occasions the fibromas may show foci of calcifications.

Q59. What is the treatment of choice in Fbroma ?
Ans. Surgical excision is the treatment of fibroma.

Q60. How do you differentiate between fibroma and fibrous hyperplasia ?
Ans. Fibroma is slow growing, asymptomatic neoplasm. Whereas fibrous hyperplasia is inflammatory reaction exhibiting excessive proliferation of fibroustissue. It is usually associated with mild trauma and may regress on removal of irritant.

Q61. What are the conditions, considered in differential diagnosis of fibromas.
Ans. Fibrous hyperplasia, pyogenic granuloma, ginat cell fibroma, and papilloma can be considered in differential diagosis of fibromas.

Q62. Write clinical feature of Giant cell fibroma.
Ans. Giant cell fibroma was first described in 1974 by Weathers anc Callihan. It may occur at any age bt common in younger age group. Clinically it appears usually as small raised, pedunulated rowth with smooth surface. It is invariably asymptomatic. The most common site of occurrence is giniva, tongue, palate, buccal mucosa and lips.

Q63. Describe the microscopic picture of Giant cell fibroma.

Ans. The microscopic picture shows presence of fibrous tissue abundantly interspersed with large stellate and multinucleated giant fibroblasts. These stellate cells have large vesicular nuclei, while cytoplasm is well demarcated.

Q64. What is the treatment of Giant cell fibroma ?

Ans. Surgical excision of the tumor is the treatment of choice in Giant cell fibroma. Recurrence is not common.

Q65. What is the peripheral ossifying fibroma ?

Ans. Even though ther are many clinically and histoloically similar lesions of fibrous growths, the peripheral ossifying fibroma is considered as separate entity containing fibrous tissue hyperplasia with formation of bone within.

Q66. Describe the clinical features of peripheral ossifying fibroma.

Ans. Clinically peripheral ossifying fibroma presents as well demarcated growth on gingiva. The growth may have pedenculated or sessile base. The surface usually is intact with no change in color. The growth is form in consistency. Peripheral ossifying fibroma occurs in younger age group. The lesion may occur in maxilla and mandible with equal frequency. The commoner site being anterior to molars.

Q67. Write the microscopic features of peripheral ossifying fibroma.

Ans. The bulk of the central mass is made up of large number of proliferating fibroblasts. Cellular component is predominant. Vascularity is not very prominent. Foci of calcification (ossification) are evident distributed in the mass. The lesion is covered by stratified squamous epithelium.

Q68. What is central Giant cell tumor ?

Ans. Central Giant cell tumor is benign neoplasm of aw bones characterized by presence of numberous giant cells. Even though it wass referred as central reparative giant cell granuloma, many do not agree with a term "Reparative" as the tumor exhibits more of destructive changes rather than reparative process. Central giant cell tumor may also show malignant form.

Q69. Write clinical features of cenral giant cell tumor.
Ans. Central giant cell tumor occurs predominantly in clildren or yonger age group. It shows predilection to female sex than male. Mandible is affected more often than maxilla. The tumor invariably occurs in the resion, anterior to first permanent molar. The tumor causes swelling or enlargement which may not be associated either with pain or paraesthesia. Teeth involved do not show displacement. Swelling caused by expansion of coticla plates, is hard and smooth.

Q70. How does central giant cell tumor appears in radiographs ?
Ans. As the central giant tumor is essentially a destructive lesion of bone, it presents as radiolucent area with relatively smooth border. Central area shows trabeculae and loculations. Presence of trabeculae, makes the lesion appear multilocular with small radiolucent spaces. Cortical plates appear thinned out. Roots may show external resorption.

Q71. Describe the histopathological features of central giant cell tumor.
Ans. Microscopic picture of cental giant cell tumors exhibits loose fibrillar connective tissue stroma with many interspersed proliferating fibroblasts and small capillaries. The arrangement of collagen fibers present whorled appearance. Multinucleated giant cells of varying sizes are distributed throughout the tumor. In addition, ther are usually numerous foci of old extravasated blood and associated hemosiderin pigment.

Q72. What are the diseases or conditions considered in the differential diagnosis of central giant cell tumor?

Ans. The various lesions which are to be considered in differential diagnosis with central giant cell tumor include, bony lesions of hyperparathyroidism, fibrous dysplasia, ameloblastoma and aneurysmalbone cyst.

Q73. Name a benign tumor of fatty tissue origin.

Ans. Lipoma is benign tumor originating from fat cells. These are not common in oral cavity.

Q74. Write the clinical features of lipoma.

Ans. Lipoma, bening tumor arising from fat cells is not a common tumor of oral cavity. However if found, it may occur on tongue, cheek, floor of mouth and mucobuccal folds. Mostly occurs in adults. It appears as single and smooth swelling with sessile base. Rarely it may be pedunculated. It is very soft in sonsistency. Margine are slippery. As it is covered with tin mucosa, the color appears yellowish.

Q75. What is the microscopic picture of lipoma ?

Ans. Microscopic picture of lipoma slhow a circumscribe mass fat cells in which many collagen fibers are interspersed. Blood vessels are few. The lesion is covered by a thin layer of stratified squamous epithelium.

Q76. How does the mature fat cells of lipoma differ from mature fat cells of body ?

Ans. Histologically the mature fat cells of lipoma and mature fat cells of body do not differ. The difference is mainly in metabolic ectivity. Fatty acid precursors are incorporated more rapidly in fat cells of lipoma. Lipopotein lipase activity is reduced. In individuals on starvation, the fat from normal fat deposits, gets lost. However such individuals on starvation do not loose fat from lipoma.

Q77. What is the treatment of lipoma ?
Ans. Surgical excision is the treatment of lipma. Recurrence is very uncommon.

Q78. What is the benign tumor originating from blood vessels ?
Ans. Hemangioma is the tumor arising from proliferation of blood vessels. It is considered as a hamartoma rather than a true neoplasm.

Q79. What is hamartoma ?
Ans. Hamartoma is an abnormal proliferation of tissues of structures native to the part.

Q80. Classify hemangioma.
Ans. Hemangiomas are classified as:
1. Capillary hemangioma, 2. Cavernous hemangioma, 3. Angioblastic hemangioma, 4. Racemose hemangioma, 5. Diffuse systemic hemangioma, 6. Metastasizing hemangioma, 7. Nevus venisus or Port wine stain and 8. Hereditary hemorrhagic telangiectasis.

Q81. Name the syndromes associated with hemangioma.
Ans. Hemangiomas are one of the features found in hereditary hemorrhagic telangiectasia or Rendu-Osler-Weber disease, CREST syndrome and encephalotrigeminal angiomatosis or Sturge-Weber disease.

Q82. Write the clinical features of hemangioma.
Ans. In mst of the cases the hemangiomas are present from birth, sometimes they arise at an early age. It is more common in females than males. These vascular proliferations may occur either as superficial soft tissue lesions or as central lesions of the bones.

Q83. Describe the clinical features of hemangiomas occurring in soft tissues of oral cavity.
Ans. The hemangioma of soft tissue of oral cavity appears similar to skin lesions. They are raised, flat and bluish red lesions on the oral mucosa. They are irregular in shape

and varying in size. The most common sites being lips, tongue, buccal mucosa and palate. The enlargements are compessibel.

Q84. What arethe clinical features of central hemangioma ?

Ans. Central hemangiomas occur within the jaw bones. Mandible is more often involved thn maxilla. Hemangiomas affect anterior part mostly. Central hemangiomas occur in younger individuals. These ar the destructive lesions resulting in osteorlytic changes. They are asymptomatic. Few cases present as painless swellings which appear similar to cyst. Teeth in involved region, are slightly mobile and exhibit pumping action.

Q85. Describe the microscopic picture of hemangioma.

Ans. Hemangiomas are composed of many small capillaries lined by a single layer of endothelial cells supported by connective tissue stroma. Such microscopic appearance most often resembles granulation tissue.

Certain hamangioma show large dilated blood vessels lined by thin endothelial lining. The sinusoidal spaces ar filled with blood. Such hemangioma ar referred to as cavernous hemangioma.

Q86. What is the treatment of hemangioma ?

Ans. Some of the congenital hemangiomas regress as age progresses. Various forms of treatments in cluding surgery, radiation, sclerosign agents, carbon dioxide snow and cryotheray have been advocated. The sclerosing agents include intralesional injection of sodium morrhuate.

Q87. Classify lymphangioma.

Ans. Lymphagions are classified as
1. Simple lympahngioma 2. Cavernous lymphangioma, and 3. Cystic lymphangioma or cystic hygroma.

Q88. Describe the clinical features of intraoral lymhangioma.

Ans. Majority of cases of lymphangiomas are present at birth but also may occur during first few years. Intraoral lesions mostly occur on tongue resulting in enlargement of tongue. They may also occur on buccal mucosa, lips and gingiva. Dorsal surface to tongue is most usual site. The superficial lesions appear as papillary lesions. These may be of normal color as surrounding mucosa, or may be of darker hue.

The deeper lesions appear as diffuse nodules with soft to firm consistency. Ther is considerable enlargement of tongue.

Q89. Write the microscopic feature of lymphangioma.

Ans. Lymphangioma is made up of numerous dilated lymphatics, lined by endothelial cell. Lymphatics are filled with lymph.

Q90. What are the tumors arising from cartilage ?

Ans. Chondroma and chondrosarcoma are the benig and malignant tumors arising from the cartilage.

Q91. Write the clinical features of chondroma.

Ans. Chondroma is a benign tumor of cartilage is not common in jaw bones. It may develop at any age and shows no apparent sex predilection. The chondroma usually arise as a painless and slow growing swelling of aw bone. The locations of chondroma is midline in maxilla and body, coronoid and condyloid process of mandible. The mucosa over the swelling mostly remans unaffected. Teeth in the involved area may exhibit mobility.

Q92. How does chondroma appears in radiograph ?

Ans. Radiographic features os chondroma are not characteristic. It may be seen as irregular radiolucent or mottled area in the bone. Roots of neighbouring teeth may show external resorption.

Q93. Write the histologic picture of chondroma.
Ans. Chondroma appears as mass of cartilage which may exhibit certain areas of calcification or necrosis. The cartilage cells appear small, contain single nuclei. Size and shape does not vary much. Cartilaginous tumors vary considerably from one area to ther area, so that same malignant tumors may present a appearance of benignity in few areas. Therefore it is essential to study larg area of biopsies for proper interpretation.

Q94. Does the adiotherapy help in treatment of chondroma ?
Ans. Radiotherapy is not useful in the treatment of chondroma as the cells are radioresistant.

Q95. What is the treatemtn of chondroma ?
Ans. Surgical removal is treatment of chondroma. Radical reseection may be necessary if the tumor is large.

Q96. Describe the clinical features of osteoma.
Ans. Osteoma is benign tumor arising from bone. It is a common tumor occurring in jaw bones. It is characterized by proliferation of either cancellous or compact bone. It may occur at any age however it is more likely to occur in yonger age group. It presents as well circumscribed swelling on jaw producing obvious asymmetry. The osteoma is slow growing tumor. Mostly it is asymptomatic. It is hard in consistency. Endosteal proliferation of osteoma may be present as a large lesion before external growth is seen. Multiple osteomas are one of the findings associated with Gargners syndrome.

Q97. What is soft tissue osteoma ?
Ans. The soft tissue osteoma is osteoma like calcified bodies found in soft tissues. They are very uncommon and may occur in tongue. They may occur at any age and may appear as solid nodules.

Q98. Write the differential diagnosis of osteoma.
Ans.   Various conditions considered in differential diagnosis include Tori, Garre's osteomyelitis, exostosis and enostosis.

Q99. What is sarcoma ?
Ans.   Sacroma is malignant tumor arising from connective tissue.

Q100. How do the sarcomas spread ?
Ans.   Sarcomas spread through the blood vessels. Hence they spread rapidly to distant aresas.

Q101. Write the clinical features of Fibrosarcoma ?
Ans.   Even though the fibrosarcoma may occur in any area where the fibrous tissue is present, it may show more predilection to the certain areas like skin, subcutaneous tissue and preiosteum. In oral cavity, the fibrosarcoma may occur in mandible, maxilla, cheek, lips, and maxillary sinus. It may occur mostly in fourth and fifth decade of life. Fibrosarcoma do not present a typical clinical features. They may present as rapidly growing swelling consisting of locally invasive fleshy and bulky mass which may show secondary changes like ulceration, and hemaorrhage.

Q102. What is osteosarcoma ?
Ans.   Osteosarcoma is the malignant tumor arising from bone. It can be either osteogenic or osteolytic depending on whether osteoblastic activity or osteolytic activity is seen.

Q103. Describe the clinical features of osteosarcoma.
Ans.   Osteosarcoma occurs most often in young males. Even though it is more common in long bones, it may also occur in either jaw bones. The manible exhibits more predilection than maxilla. Clinical features inlcude pain, loosening of teeth, rapidly progressing swelling, which may appear similar to inflammatory. The swelling may cause deformity, pain and bleeding.

Q104. Describe the radiographic features of osteosarcoma.

Ans. Osteogenic sarcoma appears as radiopaque lesion charcterised by irregularly and excessively formed bone spicules which appear radiating outwards. The characteristic radiographic feature is described as "sun ray" appearance.

Radiological appearance of osteolytic form of osteosarcoma is not characteristic. It may present as radiolucency of varying size.

Sometimes early radiological charnesi in osteosarcoma may be characterized by widening of periodontal space around the roots of multiple teeth. Theis is similar to a finding seen in scleroderma.

Q105. Write the microscopic features of osteosarcoma.

Ans. Osteosarcoma is characterized by the proliferation of osteopbalsts. These atypical neoplastic osteoblasts exhibits considerable variation in size and shape and show large, deeply stined nuclei. These are arranged in disorderly fashion around trabeculae of boen. In addition, new osteoid and bone formation may be seen. Vascular channels are positive findings. When these are exceptionally predominant, the term "telangiectatic" is applied to describe these.

Q106. Write the clinical features of Hodgkin's disease.

Ans. Hodgkins's disease is considered as one of the two main types of lymphomas. It is characterized by a bimodal age incidence peak. One in young adults and the second in the fifth decade of age. Both sexes are affected equally in younger age and older age group, However in older group, the onset is slow. The disease may stat as painless enlargement of one or more cervical lymph nodes. Later multiple lymph nodes may be involved. The nodes are usually firm and rubbery in consistency. Pain may develop due to pressure of enlarged lymp nodes on other structures. Other manifestations include generalized wekness, ocugh, anorexia, dyspnea, loss of weight and generalized itching of the skin.

Q107. What is the characteristic microscopic finding in lymph node of Hodgkn's disease ?

Ans. Presence of multinucleated cell known as Reed-Sternberg cell is the characteristic microscopic feature seen in hodgkin's disease. The are found along with lymphocytes.

Q108. What is Reed Sternberg cell ?

Ans. Reed Sternberge cell is considred to be malignant cell Hodgkin's disease. It is believed to be derived from B-lymphocyte. Possibility of other source like monocyte-macrophage has also been mentioned. However ultrastructure studies have suppoted lymphocytic origin.

Q109. What is multiple myeloma ?

Ans. Multiple myeloma is a neoplasm of bone arising from the bone marrow cells, which bear remarkable resemblance to plasma cell.

Q110. Write the clinical features of multiple myeloma.

Ans. Myltiple- Myeloma most often occurs in older age between 40 to 70 years. It is seen more in males than in females. It may present pain in bones, with or without obvious swelling. As ther is destruction of bone, pathological fractures are not uncommon. The disease may involve jaw bones. The mandible is more often affected than maxilla. Ramus and body of mandible are common sites. In jaw bones, the disease may cause pain, expansion of bone and loosening of the teeth.

Q111. Describe the radiologic features of multiple myeloma.

Ans. Radiographs of affected bone reveals numerous sharply demarcated and punched out radiolucent areas. These are multiple in number and of varying in size from few millimeters to few centimeters in diameter.

Q112. What is Bence-Jones protein ?

Ans. Bence Jones protein is an unusual protein found in the urine of persons suffering from multiple myeloma. The protein coagulates when urine is heated to 40-60⁰ C and disappears when the urine is boiled. This protein may also be found in urine of few leukemic patients.

Q113. Write the microscopic picture of lesions of Multiple myeloma.
Ans. The usual lesion of multiple myeloma is composed of sheets of closely packed cells resembling plasma cells. These cells are round or ovoid in shape with chromatin clumping in a "Cartwheel" pattern.

Q114. What is von Recklinghausen's disease ?
Ans. Von Recklinghausen's disease or Neurofibromatosis is a condition where in multiple tumors of nerve tissue occur. The specific cell of origin is still uncertain. However it is believed to originate from schwann cells, firoblasts and occasionally from perineural cells.

Q115. Write the clinical features of neurofibromatosis.
Ans. Neurofibromatosis affects mostly peripheral nerves. It can present two forms. One form consist of numerous sessile elevated smooth surfaced firm nodules of variable size, distributed over the skin of the face neck and extremities. In the second form, the nodules are deeper and larger.
In neurofibromatosis, there are additional manifestation like asymmetrically distributed cutaneous melanin pigmentation described as "Café-au-lait" spots.

Q116. Mention few tumors arising from salivary glands.
Ans. Pleomorphic adenoma, monomorphic adenoma, Warthin's tumor, oncocytoma, cylindroma, and mucoepidermoid carcinoma.

Q117. Plomorphic adenma is also called as mixed tumor. Why ?
Ans. The term pleoorphic adenoma is suggested by Willis. The tumor is called mixed tumor, as the tumor cells differentiate and metaplasia results in formation of fibrous, hyalinized, myxoid, chondroid or even osseous areas in the tumor.

Q118. Which are the cells of origin in pleomorphic adenoma ?

Ans. In histogenesis of plemorphic adenoma, it is believed that myoepithelial cells and reserve cells in the intercalated duct arethe cells from which the tumor may arise.

Q119. Is pleomorphic adenoma benign or malignant ?

Ans. Pleomorphic adenoma or mixed tumor can either be benign or malignant.

Q120. Write the clinical features of benign pleomorphic adenoma.

Ans. Benign pleomorphic tumor is a slow growing tumor and may grow into a large size in case of parotid gland. In case of intraoral tumor it may not grow into very large size as patients do seek treatment earlier due to difficulty in mastication and discomfort. Parotid gland is most often involved even though it may arise from minor salivary glands intraorally. It is more frequently seen infemales and more often seen in older age group above 40 years. The tumor arises as small nodule and grows to a large one. It usually does not cause any symptoms. Even in a very large size tumors, ulceration does not occur. The tumor is firm in consistency and not fixed to underlying tissues.

Q121. Describe the microscopic picture of benign pleomorphic adenoma.

Ans. The most characteristic feature of benign pleomorphic adenoma is diverse histologic picture with great variations. Some areas present cuboidal cells arranged in ductile arrangement and contain eosinophilic coagulum. In few areas tumor cells assume a stellate, polyhedral or spindle shape. Squamous epithelial cells may also be present. These exhibits typical intercellular bridges and sometimes even keratin s found. Loose myxoid material is frequently a premominant feature. Foci of cartilage like material or bone are common. The pleomorphic adenoma is well encapsulated tumor.

Q122. What is the origin of Muco-epidermoid carcinoma ?
Ans. The Muoc-epidermoid carcinoma is a malignant tumor arising from both mucous secreting cells and epidermoid type cels of salivary glands.

Q123. What are the clinical features of Muco-epidermoid carcinoma ?
Ans. Muco-epidermoid carcinoma may occur either in major salivary glands or mnor salivary glands of posterolateral zones of hard palate. The tumor appears as painless, slowly growing mass. Intraorally it rarely grows more than 5 cms. It is not encapsulated and may contain cyst like spaces filled with viscid mucoid material. The ulcerations may occur. Metastasis is common to reional lymph nodes. Distant metastasis may occur to lung, bone, brain and subcutaneous tissues.

Q124. Describe microscopic features of muco-epidermoid carcinoma.
Ans. The muco-epidermoid carcinoma is made up of mucus secreting cells, epidermoid cells and intermediate cells. These cells ar arranged in glandular or ductal pattern, sometimes showing microcyst formation.

Q125. What is the treatment of muco-epidermoid carcinoma ?
Ans. Surgery is the chief treatment modality. Howeer radiation may alos be helpful.

Q126. Name a benign tumor arising from epithelium of oral mucosa.
Ans. Papilloma is a common benign neoplasm arisin from oral epithelium.

Q127. What are the clinical features of papilloma ?
Ans. Papilloma, an epithelial benign neoplasm is charcterised by exophytic and pedunculated growth made up of numerous small finger like projections. It is small in size, most common intraoral sites being tongue, lips, buccal mucosa, and gingival, It is mostly asymptomatic.

Q128. Write the histologic fetures of papilloma.
Ans. Papilloma is mde up of amny logn, thin, finger like projections extending above the surface. Each finger like projection is made up of stratified squamous epithelium and contain central corium of thin connective tissue. The epithelium may show hyperkeratosis.

Q129. What is treatment of papilloma ?
Ans. Surgical excision of papilloma along with the base is ideal form of treatment.

Q130. Mention the condition considered in differential diagnosis of papilloma.
Ans. Focal epithelial hyperplasia, verruca wart, and keratoacanthoma can be considered in differential diagnosis of papilloma.

Q131. Name two syndromes associated with papillomatous lesions.
Ans. Papillomas are the one of the features of focal dermal hypoplasia syndrome and multiple hamartoma and neoplasia syndrome (Cowden's syndrome).

Q132. What is Keratoacanthoma ?
Ans. Keratocanthoma is a benign lesion of epithelial origin, sometimes resembling clinically and histologically carcinoma. It is not a carcinoma.

Q133. What is the etiology of Keratoacanthoma ?
Ans. Exact etiology is unknown, However genetic, viral and chemical carcinogens have been considered as etiological factors.

Q134. Write clinical features of Keratoacanthoma.
Ans. Keratoacanthoma occurs in older persons between 50 to 70 years. It occurs on exposed skin with cheeks, nose and lips being most often involved. It is uncommon on oral mucosa. The Keratoacanthoma appears as an elevated umblicated or crateriform lesion on the surface.

It measures less than a centimeter in size. It is slow growing. It may undergo spontaneous regression within few weeks by expulsion of keratin and regression of mass. It is often painless.

Q135. Write the histologic features of Keratoacanthoma.
Ans. Keratoacanthoma consists of hyperplasia of stratified squamous epithelium which grows into the underlying connective tissue. The surface is marked by hyperkeratosis with central plugging. The epithelial cells sometimes show dysplastic features. The deeper roup of cells appears to be invading resembling the carcinoma. The inflammatory cells are found in connective tissue.

Q136. What is the treatment of Keratoacanthoma ?
Ans. Keratoacanthoma is treated by surgical excision.

Q137. Which is the most common malignant tumor of epithelial origin ?
Ans. Squamous Cell Carcinoma is the most common malignant neoplasm originating from epithelial cells.

Q138. Which are the most common intraoral location of squamous cell carcinoma ?
Ans. Intraorally squamous cell carcinoma occurs most often on lips, tongue, floor of mouth, gingiva and buccal mucosa.

Q139. What are the precancerous lesions and conditions from which carcinoma can occur in oral mucosa ?
Ans. There are various precancerous lesion and conditions, which make the patient more prone for development of carcinoma. They are leukoplakia, Erythroplakia, Erosive lichen planus, submucous fibrosis, Plummer Vinson's syndrome and syphilitic glossitis.

Q140. Write the etiological factors in carcinoma.
Ans. Numerous etiological factors have been suggested in causation of squanmous cell carcinoma. These include use of tobacco, alcohol, and spicy foods. Other factors include chronic irritation, nutritional deficiency, sunlight, chronic

trauma, viruses and underlying precancerous lesions and conditions.

Q141. Describe the role of tobacco in causation
Ans. Tobacco is used in different forms. Smoking tobacco is used in the form of cigarettes, *beedis*, pipe smoking, *chutta*, *hukka* and reverse smoking. Reverse smoking is more prevalent in coastal areas of Andhra Pradesh. Smokeless tobacco is used in the fom of chewin tobacco. It is interesting to note thatonly 3% of patients with oral cancers had never smoked. Cigar and pipe smoking was found to increase therisk oforal cancer, than cigarette smoking. Chewing tobacco also is responsible of leukoplakic and erythroplakic changes and subsequently to oral cancer.

Q142. Write the cliical features of oral carcinoma.
Ans. Carcinoma of oral mucosa may present different clinical features in different locations. Mainly it may occur as exophytic rowth, ulceration and nodule with ulceration. Therefore the cliical features can be different for different locations.

Q143. Write the clinical features of carcinoma of lips.
Ans. Carcioma of lip occur in elderly persons. It is more common in lower lip than upper lip. Males are most often affected. Lip carcinoma often commences as a small area of thickening, induration and irregularity of surface. As it grows, it may either result in exophytic growth or crater like defect of ulceration. It is slo to metrastasize to lymph nodes. Lip carcinoma may grow to large fungatin mass.

Q144. Describe the features of carcinoma of tongue.
Ans. Among the inraoral sites of carcinoma, the gongue is affected in 25 to 50%. It is less common in women than men. Initially it may deveop as painless mass or ulcer. However most often occurs as fungating mass exhibiting ulceration with raised borders. The growth shows induction. Lateral surfaces are most often affected. Carcinoma may also occur on ventral surface and base of

the tongue. The lesion may become painful due to secondary infectin. Metastasis may occur early.

Q145. Describe the clinical features of carcinoma of floor of oral cavity.

Ans. Carcinoma of floor of oral cavity represents about 15% of all the oral cancers. It occurs in older ae group. Typical lesion occurs as indurated ulcer of floor of the oral cavity. Fungating orowth may be present. The invasion into depr tissues occurs causing limitations of tongue movements. Involvement of tongue affects speech. Lymph node involvement occurs early.

Q146. Wrte the clinical features of carcinoma of buccal mucosa.

Ans. Like other carcinomas, carcinoma of buccal mucosa also occurs in older age and more often in males than females. The carcinoma occurs mostly in lover half of buccal mucosa below the linea alba buccalis. The lesion is often painful. The ulceration shows deepr invasion and induration. Carcinoma of buccal mucosa causes limitation of opening of mouth.

Q147. Describe the clinical features of carcinoma of maxillary sinus.

Ans. Carcinoma of maxillary sinus is less frequent than other intraoral carcinomas. Maxillary sinus carcinoma is very dangerous disease as diagnosis is delayed most often. It often extensively spreads before patients become aware of the clinical symptoms. It is more common in males. In initial stages it is a symptomatic or it may resemble just sinustitis. Once it grows to lare size, it may cause loosening of maxillary teeth, bleeding around teeth, bulging and swelling of alveolar bone, palate. Bleeding from nose is common feature. Lateral spread may cause bulging of middle third of face Metastasis occurs very late when the cancer becomes more advanced.

Q148. What is TNM classification ?
Ans.   TNM classification is a clinical classification of malignant tumor based on their size, lymph node involvement and metastasis.

Q149. What is TNMP classification ?
Ans.   Criteria for TNMP classification considers not only their size, lymph node involvement and metastasis but also in adition histopathlogical features are considered. This classification is useful for treatment planning and prognosis.

Q150. Mention the criteria for size of tumor.
Ans.   Tumor size is classified into the following groups
   T1 - Tumor less than 2 cms in its greats diameter.
   T2 - Tumor more than 2 cms but less than 4 cms in this greatest diameter.
   T3 - Tumor greater than 4 cms in greatest diameter.

Q151. Write the criteria for determination of lymph node status.
Ans.   The following grouping is done for lmph nodes.
   No - No clinically palpable lymph node.
   N1 - Clinically palpable homolateral lymph nodes but not fixed.
   N2 - Clinically palpable contra lateral or bilateral lymph nodes, not fixed but metastasis suspected.
   N3 - Clinically palpable lymph nodes that are fixed and metastasis suspected.

Q152. Mention the stages of metastasis.
Ans.   There are two categories
   M0 - No Metastasis
   M1 - Clinical or radiographi evidence os distant metastasis

Q153. Describe clinical staging of oral carcinoma
Ans.   Stage I   T1 N0 M0
       Stage II   T2 N0 M0

Stage III	T3 N0 M0, T1 N1 M0, T2 N1 M0, and T3 N1 M0
Stage IV	T1 N2 M0, T2 M0, T3 N2 M0, T1 N3 M0, T2 N3 M0, T3 N3 M0, and any T N category with M1.

Q154. Which are the type of lymph nodes generally involved in case of oral carcinomas.
Ans. Submental, submangibular and cervical lymph nodes are involved from carcinomas of different parts of oral cavity.

Q155. What is Brober's Classification ?
Ans. Based on the microscopic picture Broder has classified oral cavity carcinomas into four grades.
Grade I Well differentiated.
Grade II Less well differentiated.
Grade III poorly differentiated
Grade IV undifferentiated.

Q156. What do you mean by term differentiation ?
Ans. The term differentiation is used to indicate as to whether the cells of carcinoma resemble the cells of epithelium and present characteristic features and behaviour of epithelial cells.

Q157. Describe the microscopic features of well-differentiated oral carcinoma.
Ans. The well-differentiated carcinoma consists of sheets and nests of epithelial cells. The cells are large and show distinct cell wall but intercellular bridges may be absent. The nuclei of the cells are large and darkly stained (Hyperchromatic nuclei). Mitotic figures may be present. Another prominent feature is keratinisation of individual cell and presence of epithelial pearls of varying size.

Q158. Describe the microscopic features of undifferentiated carcinoma of oral cavity.
Ans. Undifferentiated carcinomas bear very little resemblance to their cells of origin and often will present diagnostic difficulties because of the primitive, and uncharacteristic

histologic appearance of malignant and rapidly dividing cells. These cells show greater lack of cohesiveness and variant picture. The cells are highly anaplastic, and showed no Keratin formation at all.

Q159. Which organ may show distant metastsis from oral carcinomas ?
Ans. Distant metastasis through blood stream is uncommon in oral carcinomas. However ther have been few reports of distant metastasis of lungs, liver and bones.

Q160. What is the treatment of carcinomas of oral cavity ?
Ans. Depending upon the location, lymph node involvement and histopathological features, the treatment of oral carcinomas may include chemotherapy, surgery and radiotherapy. These procedures may be under taken in combination or otherwise.

Q161. Which form of radiation is used in the treatment of oral carcinoma ?
Ans. Radiotherapy of oral carcinoma can be undertaken either by teletherapy or by brachytherapy.

Q162. What is Teletherapy ?
Ans. Use of radiation beam from external radiation source is known as teletherapy. The radiation is given in divided repeated doses for 3-4 weeks. The total dose, which may be required, may be 60 to 6 gy. The source of radiation may be either electron beam or Cobalt 60.

Q163. What is the brachytherapy ?
Ans. Use of radiation source within the tumorous mass in brachytherpy. Thus interstitial and intacavitary implants are used. These implants include radium needles or radon needles.

Q164. How does the radiation kill the cells.
Ans. Radiations damages the cells by interaction with water moleculaes in the cells, producting hydroxyl groups and then cell destruction. It also causes chromosomal

damages, resulting either in cell destruction or incapacity to to divide further. Due to greater capacity to repair in normal cell, as compared to malignant cells, the normal cells are allowed to repair and regain by undertakin the radiotherapy in fractions.

Q165. What is verrucous carcinoma ?
Ans. Verrucous carninoma is slightly different and mild form of carcinoma. This was described by Ackermann in 1948. It is generally seen in older people. Most common sites being buccal mucosa, gingia or alveolar mucosa. Verrucous carcinoma is exophytic, superficially spreading neoplasm with appearance of papillary with white pebbly surface. The lesions commonly have rugae like folds with deep celefts between them.

Q166. Write the microscopic features of verrucous carcinoma.
Ans. Even though there is epithelial proliferation mitotic activity, pleomorphism, or hyperchromatism is at low degree. The epithelium is well differentiated. Cleft like spaces lined by parakeratin extend deeply from surface. Parakeratin plugging extending to epithelium is also characteristic feature. Basement membrane will often appear intact.

Q167. What is the treatment of verrucous carcinoma ?
Ans. Surgical excision of the lesion is mostly effective management of verrucous carcinoma.

14.

SYNDROMES OF HEAD AND NECK

The heritage of the term "syndrome" is ancient. It was used by Hippocrates to denote a group of regularly concurrent signs or symptoms that could result from several causes. The word syndrome has been used in New English Dictionary (N.E.D.) as a "Concurrence of several symptoms in a disease" or "A set of such concurrent symptoms". It is nowadays applied also to collections of signs, to mixed collections of symptoms and signs, and sometimes to a disease entity. It may even apply to special clinical test findings; or to a specific laboratory finding, as in Guillain Barre Syndrome.

So the term syndrome is used when the aggregated of signs, symptoms, or other manifestations considered to constitute the characteristics of a morbid entity; used especially when the cause is unknown. It is more commonly applied than disease to any postualated morbid entity whose characteristic are not well established.

It is curious how whimsically one choose the name rather than another to perpetuate a syndrome. Initially the name given for syndrome was that of a erson who described it (eponym). Later some effort was made to link the disease with the name of the patient rather than that of the physician. Even syndromes have been named according to the etiology, anatomic location (Oculodentodigital Syndrome), amin symptom (Progeressive hemifacial atrophy), or some other characteristics.

APERT'S SYNDROME

Synonyms
Acrocephalo syndactyly.
The syndrome consists of acrocephaly

(oxycephaly) and syndactyly.

Etiology
Although numerous theories have been proposed, none have gained general support. It seems to be transmitted as an autosomal dominant trait.

Clinical Features

Most features resemble Crouzon's syndrome
Face
Face is usually asymmetric. The middle third of the face is underdeveloped and flat, producing a relative prognathism. The nose is usually appeared as parrot's beak. Hypertelorism, exophthalmos and strabismus are aften reported.

Skull

The cranium is usually oxycephalic in appearance. The apex of the cranium is located near to or anterior to the bregma. Anterior fontanelle is open in numerous patients.

Extremities

There is syndactyly. It varies from partial fusion of the skin to a true osseous syndactyly of fngers and toes. When fingers are completely fused, ther is often a common nail, giving an appearance of thalidomide child.

Oral manifestation

High arched palate, cleft palate or bifid uvula and malocclusion have been reported.

Other findings
The majority of affected patients have an intelligence distinctly below normal. Other findings incude aplasia or ankylosis of several joints especially elbow, shoulder and hip; ankylosis of vertebrae and spina fibida. Heart malformations have alsobee nreproted.

ASCHER'S SYNDROME

Synonyms
Double lip, Blepharochalasis, and nontoxic thyroid enlargement.

Etiology
Etiology is unknown; suggested are hormonal dysfunction, trauma and heredity.

Clinical Features
Lips

There is a horizontal line running between the inner and outer parts of upper lip appearing double lip. Very rearly lower lip is also enlarge. The enlargement of lip may exist from childhood. The extra lip or the tissue is usally seen shen the patient smiles or during talking. Microscopic examination of this excessive tissue usually consists of loose areolar tissue and hyperplastic mucous glands.

Eyes
There is dooping of the tissue between the eyebrow and the edge of upper eyelid, so that it hands over the palpebral fissure. This is caused by relaxation of supratarsalfold as a result of atrophy and thining of the eyelid. The swelling of eyelids and enlargement of lip may occur simultaneously. On exa,mination the tissue contains orbital fat or hyperplastic lacrimal gland.

Thyroid
There is nontoxic thyroid gland enlargement. But this features is not constant. It may appear several years after the eyelid involvement, but usually appears during second decade.

Treatement
The excess tissue can be removed surgically.

BABY BOTTLE SYNDROME

Synonyms
Bottle mouth syndrome; Nursing bottle caries.

Etiology
It has been attributed to prolonged use of:
1. A nursing bottle containing mild or milk formula, fruite juice or sweetened water.
2. Breaste feeding.
3. Sugar or honey, sweetened pacifiers.

Usually these above mentioned are used as an aid for sleeping at night or at naptme.

Clinical Featutres
It presents as a wide spread carious descruction of deciduous teeth, most commonly the maxillary incisors, followed by first molars and then the cuspids. But the mandibular incisors spared. The reason for the mandibular incisors being spared is that, They are covered and protected by tongue, which bottle feeding.

Treatment
Early excavation of caries and restorations.

BEHCET'S SYNDROME

Synonyms
Recurrent genitor-oral aphthosis and uveitis with hypopy-on: Cutaneomucouveal syndrome; Generalised aphthosis; Adamantiades Behcet syndrome.

Etiology
Etiology is uncertain. In part it has been suggested to be caused by pleuropneumonia like organism (PPLO) or more frequently by virus. But now it is thought to be of autoimmune in origin.

Clinical Features
It usually beins between 10 to 45 years of age and is more common in males. It is characterized by oral and genital ulcerations, ocular lesions and skin lesions.

Eyes
The ocular signs usually begin in one eye and spread to the other. The lesions may vary in severity. These amy manifest as conjunctivitis, keratitis, uveitis with hypopyon, which may lead to severe visual damage and eventual blindness. Photophobia may also occur.

Genitalia
The genital lesions consist of recurren aphthae, larger than those involving the mucosa, which in males appear on the penis, the inner thigh, and particularly on scrotum.

In women the ulcers occur on the vulva. Perineum may be involved in both the sexes. Healing of these lesions may lead to severe scrring.

Skin
The skin lesions are generally small pustules or papules on the trunk or likbs. Another common finding is erythema nodosum.

Oral Manifestations
Oral lesions may be the first manifestation of the disease. The oral ulcers may eb located any where in th oral mucosa. They occur in crops which are very painful. They resemble aphthae, being well demarcated and varying in size from a few mm to cm in diameter.

The ulcers have an erythematous border and are covered by a gray or yellow exudates.

Other signs include thrombophematous border and are covered by a gray or yellow exudates.

Other signs include thrombophlebitis, arthralgia, epididymitis. Visceral involvement particularly of the lungs may also be seen.

Laboratory findings
Hypergammaglobulinemia, leukocytosis with eosinophilia and elevated erythrocyte sedimentation rate.

A new set of diagnostic criteria include – recurrent oral ulceration occurring at least 3 times in one 12 – month period plus 2 of the following 4 manifestations:-
1. Recurrent genital ulceration
2. Eye lesions includeing uveitis or retinal vasculitis
3. Skin lesions including erythema nodosum, pseudofolliculitis, papulo-pustular lesions, or acne from nodules in post adolescent patients not receiving corticosteroids.
4. Positive pathergy test.

According to Katzenellenbogen, patients showed characteristic erythematous reaction when an intracutaneous injection of saline was given.

Treatment

There is no specific treatment for the disease other than symptomatic or supportive measures. Patients with life threatening vasculitis should be managed with a combination of immunosuppressive drugs and corticosteroids. Cyclosporine in combination with corticosteroids had shown to be useful.

BRITTLE BONE SYNDROME

Synonyms

Ekman's syndrome; Lobstein's syndrome; Vorlik's syndrome: Eddowe's syndrome; Osteogenesis imperfecta.

The syndrome consists of fragile bones, blue sclera, laxity of ligaments, hearing loss and dentinogenesis imperfecta.

It is inherited as an autosomal dominant character, although it can also express as autosomal recessive charcter.

Etiology

Biochemical findings sugges that it is an inborn error of collagen metabolism. Primary defect in most cases appears to involve type 1 collagen.

Clinical Features

Musculo Skeletal System

Skull is large in anteroposterior direction and there is bulge in temporal region. The long bones are extremely fragile and porous, with a high tendency of fracture.The fracture may occur while an infant is just crawling or walking. The fractures heal readily, but the newly formed one again is of a similar imperfect type. The legs are bowed. The length of the long bones are usually normal, unless multiple fractures have caused undue shortening.

An abnormal electrical reaction of the muscles have been observed, the rate of contraction and relaxation being slow. There can be lexity of ligaments, resulting in habitual dislocations of joints.

Healing is often poor and hypertrophic scrring is common.

Eyes

Sclera is pale blue, which is due to thinning of the sclera, allowing the pigmented choroids to be transmitted.

Ear
Deafness is one of the frequent findings. Deafness usually begins in the third decade and increase with time. The deafness is due to osteosclerosis.
Oral manifestations
As there is disturbance of mesodermal tissue, it is but logical to think of dentine abnormality (dentinogenesis imperfecta). The deciduous teeth are affected in about 80% of patients and permanent teeth in only 35%. The teeth are noted to be translucent or opalescent. The colour of the teeth ranges from a gray to brownish violet or yellowish brown. The colour dakens with ae. The enamel may be lost early in incisal and occlusal surfaces, because of absence of scalloping between dentino-enamel junction.

Roentgenographic Features
The roots may be short and blunt. The pulp chamber and canals are greatly diminished in size or even totally absent.

Treatment
There is no known treatment for the syndrome.

BURNIGN MOUTH SYNDROME

Synonyms
Oral dysaesthesia: Glossodynia: Glossopyrosis stomatodynia: Stomatopyrosis.

Etiology
Many etiological factors have been suggested which include:
1. Local factos-denture irritation or sensitivity to denture base, candidiasis, bacterial infections, allergies to mercury.
2. Systemic factors-Vitamin deficiency, hormonal and immunologic disturbances, iron deficiency and side effects of drugs.
3. Psychogenic factors are lso considered to play an important role in etiology of burning mouth an important role in etiology of burning mouth syndrome.
4. Xerostomia

Clinical Features
Patients with the syndrome describe their symptoms as "a burning feeling" and the symptoms may vary from slight to severe. It can be continuous or intermittent.

Women ar more commonly involved than men in the age group between 40-49 years.

The tongue is reported to be the most frequent site, followed by alveolar mucosa, lips and cheeks.

Associated symptoms include taste disturbances, dry mouth sleep disturbances, headaches and non-speciic health problems.

The burning sensation is mostly quantified using linear analogue scales such as VAS scale.

By some authors, Burning mouth syndrome is regarded as a variant of atypical facial pain.

Treatment
It is important to diagnose and treat the underlying causes first. Removal of local irritants, antifunal angents and treatment of deficiencies is helpful.

Symptomatic relief is obtained from the use of topical analgesics such as 0.5% aqueous diphenhydramine alone or mixed with 0.5% dyclomine or lidocaine or other analgesic ointments applied to the affected area.

CANDIDIASIS ENDOCRINOPATHY SYNDROME

Etiology
Etiology is obscure. It is transmitted as autosomal recessive trait

Clinical Features
The syndrome consists of chronic mucocutaneous candidiasis and presence of one or more autoimmune endocrinopathies, particularly hypoparathyroidism and / or Addison's disease. Chronic lymphocytic thyroiditis, pernicious anemia, diabetes mellitus are other immunological related disorders. The candidal infection usually occurs in the first few years of life and precedes the endocrine problems by upto 13 years. Candidiasis is relatively mild and is usually restricted to oral cavity and finger nails (Especially thumb nails). Other mucosal surfaces like esophagus, oropharynx, larynx and vagina can also be involved. There can also be candida induced strictures of oropharynx and esophagus which can cause dysphagia, and hoarseness of voice.

A variety of immunologic abnormalities have been reported mainly those affecting the cell mediated immune system. It has been also reported that there is a specific inability to respond to antigens of candida albicans, so that delayed hypersensitivity and / or production of lymphokines can be mpaired or absent.

Treatemnt

Systemic and/ or topical antifungal agents are commonly and beneficially used. Especially Nystatin and Amphotericin B are used. In addition, correction of endocrinopathies and substitution for Vitamin A and iron has also been advocated.

CHEDIAK-HIGASHI SYNDROME

It is an uncommon genetic diease, which is transmitted as an autosomal recessive trait.

There is defect in granule containing cells, such as granulocytes and melanocytes. Abnormal granules also have been observed in renal tubular cells, nerve cells, and fibroblasts. The giant melanosomes in skin and hair result in pigment dilution.

Clinical Features
Ulcerationso of the oral mucosa, severe gingivitis and glossitis are commonly reported.

Infections
There are recurrent bacterial infections of the skin and respiratory tract. The reason being abnormal granules seen in blood granulocytes results in neutrophils with decreased chemotactic and bacteriocidal ability, although phagocytosis remains intact. The abnormality in bactericidal activity is thought to be caued by an inefficient use of lysosomal enzymes.

Other Features
Hypopigmentation will be noted in skin and hair resulting from pigment dilution. Neurophathy and ataxia are prominent features in some patients. Photophobia, nystagnmus, generalized lymphdenopathy and Hepatosplenomegaly have also been reported.

Laboratory Findings
Hematologic studies show giant blue-gray granules in the cytoplasm of granulocytes. These granules are hallmark of the syndrome.

Treatment and Prognosis

Patients die of recurrent infections before the age of 10 years. Those who survive the recurrent infections experience an accelerated phase of the disease that resembles lymphoma. Ther is no specific treatment; the treatment should be supportive to control infection which are usually as a result of gram positive organisms, by antibiotics. Even bone marrow transplantation has been helpful.

COSTEN'S SYNDROME

It is a smptom complex originally described by Costen in 1934.

Etiology
The signs and symptoms of the syndrome arose because of loss of posterior teeth, resulting in over closure and altered temperomandibular joint function. The pain resulted from pressure on the chorda tympani or auruculotemporal nerves. However, subsequent investigators have failed to support this evidence.

Clinical Faeatures
Impairment of hearing, either continuous or intermittent. A stuffy sensation in the ears especially at the meal time. Tinnitus, sometimes accompanied by a snapping noise whil chewing. Otalgia, dizziness and headache appears and sometime increasing towards the end of the day. Burnign sensation in the throat, tongue and side of nose.

CREST SYNDROME

It consists of five major findings-Calcinosis cutis, Raynaud's phenomenon, esophageal hypomotiligy, sclerodactyly and telangiectasia. It is a variant of systemic sclerosis. Systemic sclerosis is characteriseded by progressive fibrosis of skin and multiple organs, and by vascular insufficiency through abnormalities in arterioles and capillaries.

This form of disease is sometimes not as severe as the systemic sclerosis. Clacinosis cutis – is ectopic calcification seen in skin. It shows foreign body rection.

Raynaud's phenomenon – is a disorder characterized by intermitten vasopastic episodes triggered by cold or emotional stimuli, resulting in ischaemia of the fingers, toes or both. Clinically it is characterized by a typical triphasic colour response, which consists of pallor, cyanosis and rubor in the same order of occurrence, involving the affected extremity.

CROUZONE'S SYNDROME

Synonyms
Craniofacial dys ostosis

Etiology
Crouzon suggested that at birth the sutures of the cranial bones were inflamed; causing premature closure of the fontanels, early bone synostosis and a latent period of cranial bone growth.

It is transmitted as an autosomal dominant trait.

Clinical Feature
Oral Manifestations

Hypoplastic maxilla, which causes a relative prognathic appearance of mandible. Theshap of the arch in "V" shaped with crowding of maxillary teeth in cuspid region. As the maxillary arch is smaller thn mandibular arch, the occlusion of mandibular teeth is often buccal and labial to maxillary teeth.

The palate is short and high arched; clefting (of either hard or soft palate) is also evident. Partial anodontia and unerupted teeth have been reported.

Face
It is characteristic. Patients show a protruberant frontal region, with an anteroposterior ridge overhanging the frontal eminence and often passing to the root of the nose (triangular frontal object). The patients nose is described s resembling parrot's beak.

Cranium

The cranium is brachioc, with shortening of an terposterior length and widening of transverse diameter of the skull.

Roentgenographically, the coronal, saittal and lamdoid sutures are prematurely synostosed. In half of the cases, ther is widening of pituitary fossa.

Eyes
Exopthalmus is a constant and characteristic feature. This might be due to increased intracranial pressure. Hypertelorism, nystagmus have been reported. The mentality of the patent may or may not be retarded.

Treatment
Cranectomy at a very age to provide space for rapidly developing brain has been used. In past few years, sophisticated surgical procedures have been developed to improve cosmetic appearance and vision of patients.

CUSHING'S SYNDROME

Cushings syndrome can be defined as the symptoms and signs associated with prolonged exposure to inappropriately elevated levels of plasma corticosteroids.

Etiology
The patients can be divided into two main groups:
1. ACTH dependent causes of Cushing's Syndrome
2. Non-ACTH dependent causes of the syndrome

1. *ACTH dependent causes*
    - Latrogenic – Administration of excessive quantities of ACTH or its synthetic analogues.
    - Pituitary – dependent bilateral adrenocortical hyperplasia.
    - Ectopic ACTH syndrome – secretion of ACTH by benign or malignant tumors of non-endocrine origin.

2. Non-ACTH dependent causes
    - Latrogenic – administration of supra physiological doses of corticosteroids.

- Adenomas or carcinomas of the adrenal cortex. When ther is bilateral adrenocortical hyperplasia conventionally it is called as Cushing's disease. Cushing's disease represents approximately 75% of the causes of Cushing's syndrome.

Clinical Features
It is more common in females in the age group of 35-50 years.

The most striking feaures is rounded plethoric face "moon face", cental obesity and "buffalo hump" due to accumulation of fat at lower parts of the back of the neck.
Other features incude, glycosuria not controlled by insulin.
Recession of hair on forehead, weakness, easy bruising and purple striae of skin over he abdomen, buttocks and thighs. It can produce back ache, yphosis, and shortening of stature. These are as a result of osteoporosis.

Intraoral Manifestation
Pigmentation may be present at any site of oral cavity. The gingiva, buccal mucosa and palate may be blotchy.

Treatemnt

Bilateral adrenalectomy preceded by the control of adrenocortical function with metyrapone.
DOWN'S SYNDROME

Synonyms
Trisomy 21; Mongolism; G trisomy.

It is a disease associated with subnormal mentality in which as extremely side variety of anomalies and functional disorders may occur; two of the chief types being cranial and facial deformities.

Etiology
Many factors, such as advanced maternal age and ulterine and placemental abnormalities, have been regarded as causes. Recent investigations now implicate a chromosomal aberration.

Incidence

This is the most common chromosomal abnormality to occur in man. The incidence is approximately 1-2 per 1000 births.

Types
Ther are at least 3 forms of Down syndrome.
One- in which ther is typical trisomy 21 with 47 chromosomes.

Second- translocation type, in which only 46 chromosomes are present, although the extra chromosome material of number 21 is translocated to another chromosome of G or D group of chromosome 13 or 15.

Third – is result of mosaicism, (three types of mosaicsm, cellular mosaicism, tissue mosaicism and chimerism). The syndrome may be seen in association with Klinefelters syndrome (XXY) and / or in relation to eukemia.

Clinical Features

Oral Manifestations

Open mouth is common finding. Tongue is large fissureing and furrowing and enlargement of papilla have been noted. Lips are broad, irregular, fissured and dry. Palate is high arched and it is also reported that mandible is "V" shaped. Maxillary lateral incisor is abnormal in 35% of patients, and can be missing or peg shaped. Periodontal bone loss is severe, even below the age of six years, especially inlower anterior reion. Surprisingly, these patients had a very low caries incidene. Narcotizing ulcerative gingivitis is common in this syndrome.

Other Features

Flat face, lare anterior fontanel, open sutures, small slanting eyes with epicanthal folds, strabismus, bystagemus, cataract, short nose, brachycephaly, short stature, poor development of bones of middle face, producing relative prognathism. Actually the defects are so varied in their occurrence that is is difficult to make a complete list.

Cardio Vascular Anomalies

Congenital cardiac problems are present in 40% of infants with Down syndrome which includes-ventricular septaldefect, arterio-venus communis, arterial septal defect, patent ductus arteriosus, and mitral valve prolapse.

Hematopoietic Anomalies

Impaired immunity like defectie short lived neutrophils, risk of lymphopenia, impaired cell mediated imunity, and irregularserum immunoglobulin patterns. Patients are at greater risk of developing leukemia, approximately 1 in 200 is affected. There is 7 times greater probability of being a carrier of hepatitis virus than general population.

Musculo Skeletal

Atlanto axial instability and under development of mid face with relative prognathism.

Nervous System Anomalies

Dementia, delayed motor functions and delay in expressive language.

EAGLE'S SNDROME

Synonyms

Stylohyoid syndrome; Stylalgia.

The disorder is due to an elongated styloid process and/or calcification of stylohyoid or stylomandibular ligament. The styloid process is considred elongated when the total length of the bony process and/ or the mineralized portion of one of the ligaments exceeds 30 mm on the radiograph. (The normal length of the styloid process is 20-25 mm.).

Classification:

Type 1 Elongated – Radiographic appearance is characterized by an uninterrupted integrity of styloid image.

Type 2 pseudoarticulated – Styloid process is apparently joined to the mineralized stylomandibular or stylohyoid ligament, by a single pseudo articulation, which is located superior to a level tangential to the inferior border of mabdible.

Type 3 Segmented – it consists of either short or long noncontinuous portions of the styloid process or interrupted segments of mineralized ligament. In either instance two or more segments are seen with interruptions either above or below the level of inferior border of the mandible.

Clinical Features

The first syndrome consists of typical complant "as if a sharp foreign body is lodged in the throat". This results in pain when swallowing and the tendency to swallow more often than normal in an attempt to get rid of the object. The pain is described as deep and dull in the region of oropharynx and posterior auricular reion. There is limited range of neck motion.

The second syndrome called the "carotid artery Syndrome", is caused by mechanical irritation of the sympathetic nerve tissue in the walls of the internal and/or external carotid artery, by the tip of the styloid process or the ossified ligament. This impingement produces referred pain in the respective area of vascularisation. In case of involvement of the external carotid artery, the pain will be related to the intraorbital and/ or temporal regions and/or the ear or occiput areas. The patient may also complain of tinnitus, otalgia and pain on turning the head. When the internal carotid artery is triggered, complains of pain in the distribution area of ophthalmic artery and in the parietal region.

Diagnosis

Radiographs show elongated styloid process (that is more than 30 mm) and increased pain during sallowing and following intraoral lateral pharyngeal palpation.

Treatemnt

Simple fracturing of the process and surgical shortening by intraoral approach.

ELLIS-VAN CREVELD SYNDROME

Synonyms

Chondroectodermal dysplasia: Mesoectodermal dysplasia.

The syndrome appears to be inherited as an autosomal recessive trait. About 25% of the atients have parental consanguinity and bout 25% of affected persons have had affected siblings.

Clinical Features

Facies
It is not characteristic, except for a mild defect in the middle of the upper lip.

Extremities and Other Skeletal Anomalies
The extremities ar often plump and markedly shortened progressively distal ward, that is form trunk to the phalanges. Bilateral manual hexadactyly is frequent, the extra digit being on the ulnar side. The fibula is most severely shortened, being only about 50% of normal length. Phalangeal bones are often missing.

Heart
Congenital heat defect is not a constant feature, it has been only in 50-60% of cases. The most common defect demonstated was interseptal defect, some patients have had cortriloculare.

Hair and Nails
The eye brows and pubic hair, have been stated to be thin and sparse. Severe dystrophy of nails can be seen. They are markedly hypoplastic, thin and often wrinkled or spoon shaped.

Eyes
The eyes are usually normal but internal strabismus, congenital strabismus and coloboma of the iris have been observed.

Genitalia
About 1/3rd of patients are noted to have genital anomalies.

Mental Status
About 1/3rd of patients are noted to be mentally retarded.

Oral Manifestations
The most constant oral finding is fusion of the middle portion of the upper lip of the maxillary ginival margin, so that no mucobuccal fold or sulcus exists anteriorly. Because of this fusion, the milled portion of the upper lip appears hypoplastic, resembling a lip that has undergone cheiloplasty.

Natal teeth, prematurely erupted deciduous teeth frequently occur. There is often deficiency in number of teeth especially in the lower anterior region. In this region the alveolar ridge is often serrated. Tooth eruption is often delayed and those erupted are usually small, conical and irregularly palced. The enamel has been noted to be hypoplastic.

Treatment
There is no treatment for the disease. Some patients die early in childhood.

FREY'S SYNDROME

Synonyms
Auriculotemporal syndrome; Gustatory sweating; Dupuy's syndrome.

Etiology
There is damage to auriculotemporal nerve and subsequent re-innervation of sweat gland by parasympathetic salivary fibers.

The syndrome usually follows some surgical operations such as removal of partid tumor or the ramus of mandible or a parotitis of some type that has damaged the auriculotemporal nerve. After a considerable time following surgery, during which the damaged nerve regenerates, the parasympathetic salivary nerve supply develops innervating the sweat glands, which then function after salivary, sustatory or psychic stimulation.

Other theories have been proposed; among them denervation hypersensitivity i.e. hypersensitivity of the skin of the affected area to acetylcholine released from the salivary gland, has gained lot of omportance. Other appear due to transaxonal excitation rather than to actual autonomic misdirection of fibres.

Clinical Features

Patient typically exhibits flusing and sweating of the involved side of face, chiefly in the temporal area, during eating. Profuse sweating may be evoked by parental administration of pilocarpine or eliminated by administration of stropine. As a rule, once the syndrome appears the area of the skin involved increases in size.

Related to auriculotemporal syndrome is the "chorda tymkpani" syndrome. In this syndrome the sweating and flushing are limited to the skin of the chin and submental region. This is usually rare and may accompany operation or injury to the submandibular gland.

Treatment
Intracranial division of the auriculotemporal nerve has been reported to be successful.

GARDERNERS'S SYNDROME

Synonyms

Multiple osteomas; Fibrous and fatty tumors of the skin and mesentery; Epidermoid inclusion cysts of skin and multiple intestinal opolyposis.

It has been suggested that the syndrome is transmitted as an autosomal dominant trait with marked penetrance and variable expressivity.

Clinical Features
Skin and Appendages
Skin if frequently the site of epidermoid inclusion cysts. These may appear any where on the face, trunk or extremities. Occasionally fibromas and desmoids, may occur.

Gastrointestinal Disorders

Multiple intestinal polyposis of colon and rectum, with a marked tendency to rapid malignant transformation is characteristic.

Fibromas and fibrosarcomas may be found scattered through out the mesentery.

Oral Manifestation

Multiple osteomas may be scattered throughout the calvarium and facial skeleton and occur frequently on frontal, maxillary and mandibular bone. Numerous multiple impacted supernumery teeth and permanent teeth are present.

GORLIN AND GOLTZ SYNDROME

Synonyms

Jaw cysts – Basal cell nevus – Bifid rib syndrome; Basal cell nevus syndrome; Hereditary cutaneomandibular polyoncosis.

It is transmitted as an autosomal dominant trait.

Clinical Features

Cutaneous Anomalies

Multiple nevoid basal cell carcinomas usually appear about puberty. Nose, upper eyelids, cheeks, trunk, neck, are commonly involved, however any part of skin can be involved. Cysts of skin, palmer pitting, palmer and plantar keratosis and dermal calcinosis have also been noted.

Skeletal Anomalies

1. Rib anomalies are common- bifid rib, it can involve one rib or more than one rib and can be bilateral.
2. Fusion of vertebrae and shortened fourth metacarpals have been noted
3. Mandibular prognathism is seen in several patients.

Eye Anomalies

Include hypertelorism with wide nasal bridge, dystopia canthorum, congenital cataract, glaucoma, congenital blindness nad internal strabismus.

Neurologic Anomalies

Includes mental retardation or schizophrenia, calcification of dura mater, agenesis of corpus callosum and congenital hydrocephalus.

Sexual Abnormalities

Includes hypogonadism and ovarian or uterine calcifications.

Oral Manifestation

Numerous odontogenic kerotocysts are scattered throughout the jaws varying in size from micropic to several centimeters. The cyst may appear as early as 7-8 years of age or at third decade of life. If the cysts develop early in life, there is deformity and displacement of developing teeth.

Treatment
Cyst should be surgically excised, but cyst associated with this syndrome appears to have high recurrence rate.

GRINSPAN'S SYNDROME

An association has been described between oral lichen planus, diabetes mellitus and hypertension. This triad is referred to as Grinspan's syndrome. Originally described by Grupper. But however no direct inter relationship of the three factors would appear to have been elucidated.

Christensen and his co-workers conducted a study on group of 120 patients with oral lichen planus. They neither could find, hypertension nor diagetes mellitus.

Studies have also shown that the patients receiving treatment for diabetes mellitus and hypertension, subsequently developed lichenoid reactions in oral mucosa.

Subsequent investigations of other series of patients with lichen planus have not confirmed Grinspan;s finding, other than that a proportion of patients with chronic oral problems will be found to hve diabetes and hypertension.

The exact etiology is unknown, however numerous factors have been mentioned to aggrevate or precipitate oral lichen planus such as immunologic, allergy, psychosomatic and heamotoligic.

Clinically oral lichen palnus can appear in various forms viz (a) Reticular, (b) Bullous, (c) Vesicular, (d) Ulcerative, (e) Erosive type, (f) Plaque type.

HEERFORDT'S SYNDROME

Synonyms

Uveoparotitic paralysis; Uveoparotitis;
Uveoparotid fever; Sarcoidosis.

It was described By Heerfordt, an ophthalmologist in 1909.

The etiology is unknown. But it is considered by most investigators to be a form of sarcoidosis; in which there is parotid enlargement, inflammation of uveal track and facial palsy. It effects persons in their second to third decades of life.

Clinical Features

Prodronal symptoms may arise a few days to several months prior to the appearance of the syndrome. These may include weakness, cough, polyuria, dry mouth, gastrointestinal distress, joint pain and mild fever.

Oral Manifestations

Parotid glands enlarge bilaterally, though occasionally there may be unilateral enlargement. This is usually the first sign of the syndrome. The glands are firm, nodular and painless, and never suppurate. The salivary flow rate is decrased.

Other Manifestations

Eye

Uveitis, although may being unilaterally, it eventually becomes bilateral and may cause permanent visual impairment. Iris nodules are seen in about 1/3rd of patients.

Nerveous System

The most common neurologic finding is facial paralysis (30-50%). It is bilateral in about 1/3rd cases. The palsy usually follows enlargement of parotid glands. Other cranial nerves may also be involved. Paralysis of soft palate and vocal cords have been noted. Ther is also loss of deep reflexes and polyneuritis.

Diagnosis

Microscopic examnation of involved salivary gland shows characteristic sarcoid tissue. The acini are atrophic and displaced by numerous military, partly confluent, epithelioid, caseating tubercles.

Kviem test is positive in about 85% of cases with active sarcoidosis.

Treatment

Treatment of the disease is largely symptomatic, because more than 50% of patients are either asymptomatic or have undergone spontaneous remission. Pationes who are symptomatic or suffer active inflammatory disease, corticosteroids ar dug of choice. Patients often improve symptomatically in 2 weeks but therapy should be continued for a minimum of 6-8 months.

HORNER'S SYNDROME

Synonyms

Sympathetic Ophthalmopelgia

The exact features of the syndrome depend on degree of damage of sympathetic pathways to the head and the site of the damage. Thus lesion in the brain stem, (chiefly tumors on infections) or in the cervical or high thoracic cord, occasionally produce this syndrome. Preganglionic fibres in the anterior spinal roots to the sympathetic chain in the low cervical and high thoracic area are commonly involved by infection, trauma or pressure as by aneurysms or tumor to produce the syndrome. It is characterized by-miosis or contraction of pupil of eye due to paresis of the dilator of pupil, ptosis, or drooping of the eyelid due to paresis of smooth puscle elevator of upper eyelid, and anhidrosis and vasodilation over face control due to interruption of pseudomotor and vasomotor.

HORTON'S SYNDROME

Synonyms

Sphenopataine Neuralgia, Sluder's syndrome; Atypical facial neuralgia; Cluster headache; Vidian nerve neuralgia; Periodic magranous neuralgia.

It is a pain syndrome originally described by Sluder. Men are effected more commonly than women and it occurs before the age of 40 years.

Etiology

Exact cause is unknown. It is thought to be due to,

Vasonstriction of vessels supplying the nasal mucosa.
Deviation of the nasal septum or of a septal spur causing irritation of sphenopalatine ganglion.
Irritation or inflammation of vidian nerve in the vidian canal, secondary to sphenoid sinus infection.
Widely accepted evidence currently is that is caused by vasodilation involveing the internal maxillary artery, particularly that portion supplying the sphenopalatine region.

Clinical Features

It is characterized by unilarteral paroxysms of paroxysms of intense pain in the region of eyes, the maxilla, the ear, and mastoid, base of the nose and neneath zygoma. Sometimes the pain extends into occipital area as well.

There is no trigger zone. Paroxysms of pain have a rapid onset, persists for 15 mins to several hours and then disappear as rapidly as they began.

In some patients the onset of paroxysms occur at exactly the same time of the day and for this reason, it is also referred to as "alarm clock" headache.

Other Clinical Featurs

Sneeizing, swelling of nasal mucosa and severe nasal discharge, epiphora or watering of the eyes and blood shot eyes. Paraesthetic sensations of the skin over the lower half of the face also are reported.

Treatment

Numerous methods of treatment are employed but none are successful. Most widely used is cocainization of sphenoplatine ganglion or alcohol, resection of ganglion, ergotamine has also been employed.

JAMES RAMSAY HUING'S SYNDROME

Synonyms
Geniculate ganglion syndrome; Hunt's syndrome.

It is a special form of Heres-Zoster infection of geniculate ganglion (or sensory ganglion of facial nerve).

Clinical Features

Facial paralysis as well as pain of the external auditory meatus and pinna of the ear. Vesicular eruptions occur in the oral cavity and oropharynx with hoarseness of voice, tinnitus, vertigo, loss of taste and decreased salivation. The apin is of severe type and occurs in paroxysm. Associated symptoms can be diminished hearing, vertigo, nystagmus, loss of superficial and deep sensation of face.

Treatment

Antiviral drugs such as acyclovir 800 mg 5 times a day for 10 to 14 days reduces durations of pain significantly. Patients who do not respond to medication may undergo surgery to section the nevus intermedius.

JAW WINKING SYNDROME

Synonyms

Marcus Gunn phenomenon; Pterygoid – Levator synkinesis; Corneocmandibular reflex.

It consists of unilateral congenital ptosis and rapid exaggerated elevation of the ptotic lid on moving the lower jaw to contralateral side.

Etiology

Exact cause is unknown, but numerous theories have been put forward. The most widely accepted on is that, ther is aberrant innervation of the Levator palpebraesuperioris from the motor brance of the trigeminal nerve, because of the close approximation of the nuclei of the third and fifth cranial nerves. However, a supranuclear involvement has been suggested and the view has gained support. There appears to be some hereditary pattern. The syndrome may also begin later in life, following an injury or disease.

Clinical features

It appears that males are affected more commonly than females, and the left upper eyelid is involved more frequently. The ptosis is congeenitla in over 90% of cases however it may occur in later part of the life. About 40% of the patients manifest the syndrome both on depressing the mandible and on moving it to the opposite side of the ptotic eye. Another 40% only need the jaw to be depressed. However, in some individuals, movement of lips, whistling, clenching the teeth or puffing out the cheeks may produce the syndrome.

LAZY LEUKOCYTE SYNDROME

It was first described by Miller, Oski, and Harris in 1971.

It is caused by loss of chemotactic function of neutrophils. The bone marrow contains normal numbers of mature neutrophils, but the patients have severe neutropenia because the cells are unable to migrate from the narrow to the peripheral blood. Although, phagocytic and bactericidal functions remain intact.

Clinical Features
The manifestations become apparent at the age of 1 to 2 years, when infectious complications begin. The most common infections noted are gingivitis, stomatitis, otitis media and bronchitis. It is also frequently associated with periodontal disease.

Disgnosis
The diagnosis is based on neutrophil mobilization tests, showing lack of normal respoinse to epinephrine and piromen.

MARFAN'S SYNDROME

Synonyms
Marfan-Achard syndrome; Dolichostenomelia;
Arachnodactyly; Dystrophia mesodermalis congenital.
     It is a hereditary disease transmitted as an autosomal dominant trait (Abraham Lincoln was affected). It is basically a disease of connective tissue, related to defective organization of collagen.

Clinical Features

Oral Manifestation

High arched palatal vault is very prominent and may be a constant finding. Cleft palate and bifid uvula has also been reported. In addition, multiple odontogenic cysts of maxilla and mandible have occasionally been reported.

OIther Manifestions

Facies

The head is usually dolicocephalic, with prominent supraorbital ridges and a long thinface which commonly suggests the diagnosis of the disease. Frontal bossing is common, and the eyes often appear sunken. The ears are often large, with an abnormally thin helix.

Cutaneous and Musculoskeletal Systems

The extremities are disproportionately long. Excessive length of tubular bones results in dolichostenomelia or disproportionately long thin extremities and arachnodactyly or spidery fingers.

Lower segment (pubis to sole) is greater than the upper segment (vertex to pubis). Normally the upper to lower segment ratio is 0.93 (in white adult). Hyper extensibility of joints with habitual dislocations, Kyphosis or scoliosis and flat foot are other features.

Eyes
Bilateral ectopia lentis caused due to weakened or brokens suspensory ligaments is presents in at least 50% of patients. Myopia is usually present. In addition the lens may be abnormally small and spherical.

Cardiovascular System

Diffuse dilation of ascending aorta, dissecting aneurysm, both may occur and are preceded by aortic regurgitation inat lease 65% cases.

Laboratory Aids
- Determination of upper to lower segment ratio.
- Low serum mucoprotein level and high urinary hydroxyproline level.

Treatment
No specific treatment and the prognosis is good.

MELKERSSON – ROSENTHAL SYNDROME

Synonyms

Melerson syndrome; Miescher's syndrome; Recurrent edema bound granulomatosis. The maority of investigators have considered Melkersson Rosenthal syndrome as identical with Miescher's chelitis granulomatosa; however others have denied the relationship, because they consider chelitis granulomatosa to be a result of recurrent streptococcal infection. So, Mescher's syndrome involves diffuse swelling of lips, which is soft and exhibits no pitting upon pressure. Where as in Melkersson Roseenthal syndrome it also exhibits facial paralysis and a folded or plicated to tongue.

Etiology

Etiology is unknown, but can be hereditary or familial. Causes like infections and allergy, have also been recommended.

Clinical Features

Oral Manifestations

Buccal mucosa is swollen and is cushion like and divided by furrows of varying depth. The mucosa may be red, and tongue papilla may be atrophic. Swelling of ingiva and palate has also been reported. Floded tongue (lingua plicata) is seen in 1/3rd of patients. Sometimes the tongue changes consists only of a deepened median fissure.

Other Manifestations

Facies

Swelling of the lips either unilaterally or bilaterally is the dominant feature. The swelling begins suddenly, in most cases prior to, but sometimes after orsimulataneously with the facial paralysis. It has been observed that the swelling developed after exposure to cold weather. Uaually the upper lip is affected, but swelling of lower lip is also seen. The edema may assume a peculiar reddish-brown appearance. It is non tender and non pitting.

Eyelids, chin and nose may also be affected.

Facial paralysis begins in children or persons less tan 20 years of age. Paralysis is peripheral and clinically indistinguishable from Bel's palsy.

Histoloical Features

Granulomatous changes have been characterized by tuberculoid or sarcoi granulomas in lamina propria. The granulomas may show presence of inflammation in varyin degrees and giant cells of the Langhans type, perivascularly.

Treatment

These lesions are usually treated with topical, intra lesional and systemic corticosteroids, with surgical reduction of the lip wen the persistent swelling is a cosmetic offunctional problem.

MYOFASCIAL PAIN-DYSFUNTION SYNDROME

Synonyms

Myofascial pain-dysfunction syndrome, Masticatory myalgesia syndrome. The concept of Costen's syndrome based on occlusal disharmony with resultant damage to the temperomandibular joint causing a wde variety of signs and symptoms has now been discarded. The studies of Schwartz have shown that, its not the occlusal disharmony which causes the problem, but the entire masticatory apparatus dysfunction which is the reason, and the disease was subsequently designated as myofacial pain dysfunction syndrome (MPDS).

Etiology

The principle factor responsible for the manifestations of this syndrome is masticatory muscle spasm. This muscle spasm can be initiated as a result of muscular overextension, muscular overcontraction of muscle fatigue.

Muscular overextension may be produced by either dental restorations or prosthetic applicances which encroach on the intermaxillary space. Musuclar overconttraction may result from over closure as a result of bilateral loss of posterior teeth or continued resorption of alveolar bone after construction of a prosthetic appliance.

However most common cause appears to be muscle fatigue caused by chronic oral clenching of theteeth. This in trun may result from irritating factors, such as an overhanging margin of a restoration. These habits are believed to be involuntary, tension relieving mechanism. Thus, this explanation of the syndrome has been termed the psycho-physiologic theory by *Laskin.*

Clinical Features

More commnly females are involved, usually below the age of 40 years. Ther are four cardinal signs and symptoms of the syndrome-

1. Pain
2. Muscule tenderness
3. Clicking or popping noise in the temperomandibular joint.
4. Limitation of jaw motion, unilaterally or bilaterally.

Patients also have two negative characteristics-

1. An absence of cliical, radiographical or bio-chemical evidence of oranic changes in the joint it-self.
2. Lack of tenderness in the joint when it is palpated through the external auditory meatus.

The pain is usually unilateral and is described as a dull ache in the ear or preauricular area which may radiate to the angle of mandible, temporal or lateral cervical area. Tederness in masticatory musculature, especially lateral pterygoid followed by masseter, temporalis and medial pterygoid.

Treatemnt

To relieve the symptoms, it is essential to treat the emotional and physical components of the disorder. Using only practitioner suggestion and placebo drugs, splints or occlusal equilibration, Goodman, Greene and Lasin have shown 40% - 60% success in relieving pain.

Initial treatment and recommendations include-

- Spray and strecthc-Fluromethane refrigerant spray can be applied to the skin overlying the involved muscles. This allows patient to slowly stretch the muscles in spasm. At home, the patient can apply ice for 10 min, stretching, then placing a hot, moist compress over the area. Repeating this procedure thrice daily is often beneficial.

- Injecting local anaesthetic not containing epinephrine in trigger points of muscles of spasm.

- Soft diet.

- Asprin or any non-sterodal anti inflammatory drugs.

- Diazepam 2 mg trice daily and 5 mg at bedtime for 2 weeks.

- Transcutaneous electrical nerve stimulation (TENS) has also been beneficial.

- Acupuncture- has been used in treatment, of chronic cases.

-

ORO-FACIAL – DIGITAL SYNDROME

Synonyms

Orodigitofacial dysostosis, OFD syndrome, Dysplasia linguofacialis. According to Papillon-Leage and Psaume, the condtion is limite to females and it was an incomplete recessive trait.

Gorlin et al. believed the condition was X-Linked dominant, limited to females and lethal in males.

Clinical Features

Oal Manifestations

Clefts associated with hyperplasia of the frenula are the most striking feature. Ther is usually a small midline cleft in the upper lip extending through the vermilion border. With this pseudocleft, a wde thickened or hyperplastic reduplicated frenum is seen.

The palate is cleft laterally, deep bilateral grooves extending medially from the maxillary buccal frenum, divide the palate into a premaxillary portion containing central and lateral incisors and tow lateral palatal processes. The soft palate is often completely and asymmetrically cleft.

Numerous thick fibrous bands are present in the lower mucobucal fold, eliminating the sulcus, clefting the lower ridge and by extension bifurcating, trifurcating or tetrafurcating the tongue. Malposition of maxillary canine teeth and infraocclusion is common. Absence of mandibular lateral incisor was also observed, which might be due to thick fibrous bands.

Other Manifestations

Facies

Dystopia canthorum (lateral displacement of the cnathi), a pseudo cleft in the midline of upper lip.

Digits

Malformation of digits, including syndactyly, clinodactyly, and extra digits has been reported. In these patients degree of mental retardation seems to be exceedingly mild.

OSLER-RENDU-WEBER SYNDROME

Synonyms

Hereditary Hemorrhagic Telangiectasia; gold Steins Heredo Famialial Angiomatosis; Familial Hemorrhagic Telangiectasia.

Etiology

The disease is a cascular anomaly, the cause of which is obscure. It is thought to be transmitted as an autosomal dominant trait.

Clinical Features

The telangiectasia in this syndrome may vary in appearance.

Osler describe 3 types:

- Pinpoint
- Spider like
- Nodular

The lesions are bright red, violaceous or purple in color.

Oral Manifestations

The letangiectasia appear on vermilion border, lips, gingiva, buccal mucosa, palate; rarely, floor of the mouth and tongue are also ivolved.

      Hemorrhage from gingia and buccal muocsa occurs less frequently than from the lips and tongue.

Other Manifestations

Skin

Telangiectasia commonly occurs on the skin of face and les frequently on scalp, figners, toes and nail bed. Usually they appear in second and third decade of life.

Nasal Mucosa
Telangiectasia of nasal mucosa is common and give rise to recurrent epistaxis. As a rule epistaxis precedes the appearance of telangiectasia on the skin.

Pathology

The disease is primarily due to the defects in the small blood vessels of skin and mucosa. The actual cause is either a primary intrinsic defect of the endothelial cells permitting their detachment, or a defect in the perivascular supporting tissues.

Treatment

There is no treatment for the disease but spontaneous hemorrhages may be controlled by pressure packs, particularly nasal bleeding.

PAPILLON-LEFEVER SYNDROME

Synonyms

Palmer-plantar hyperkeratosis.

It is inherite as an autosomal recessive trait. In several cases there has been evidence of parental consanguinity.

Clinical Features

Oral Manifestations

The development and eruption of deciduous teeth proceeds normally, but almost simultaneously with the appearance of palmar and plantar hyperkeratosis. The gingiva swells and become boggy. Deep pockets are frequently present. Desctructions of periodontium follows almost immediately after the eruption of last molar tooth. The teeth are involved in roughly the same order in which they erupt. By age of 4 years, nearly all primary teeth are lost. Bony destruction is usually severe and the alveolarprocess is often completely destroyed.

Other Manifestations

Skin

The characteristic skin lesions consists of keratotic lesions of the plamar and plantar surfaces. The palms and soles become red and scaly.

In addition some patients manifest a generalized hyperhidrosis, very fine hair and a peculiar dirty colored skin. Calcification of the falx cerebri or dura is also frequently reported.

Treatment

No specific treatment. Prognois of the teeth is hopeless.

PERRY-ROMBERG SYNDROME

Synonyms

Facial hemiatrophy; Romber syndrome.

Etiology

Is unknown. It s thought to be due to trophic malfunction of the cervical sympathetic nervous system, trauma, infection, heredity, peripheral trigeminal ceuritis, form of localized scleroderma and cerebral disturbance of fat metabolism.

Clinical Features

Face

There is progressive atrophy of some or all the tissues on one side of the face, occasionally extending to other parts of the body.

The onset of the condition is usually noticed in first or second decade of life as a white line, furrow or mark on one side of the face near the midline.

This initial lesion extends progressively to include subcutaneous tissue, muscle and bone resulting in facial atrophy. The two halves of the face appear as though made up of two different individuals. Ther may be hollwing of cheeks, and the eye may appear depressed in the orbit (enophthalmic). The cartilage of nose, ear, larynx and palpebral tarsus may also become involved. Affected skin often becomes darkely pigmented. Usually left side of the face is more commony affected.

Central Nervous System

Epilepsy is most frequently reported, although, trigeminal neuralgia, facial nerve palsy, migraine headache, mental disorders ar as well reported.

Oral Manifestations

Hemiatrophy of lips and tongue is reported. Eruption of the teeth may be delayed on the involved side. The roots may exhibit deficiency of root development and reduced growth of the jaws on the affected side.

Treatment

No specific treatment. Augmentation of the atrophic areas for esthetic improvement and symptomatic treatment for neurological disorders can be doen.

PEUTZ-JEGHERS SYNDROME

Synonyms
Hereditary intestinal poyposis; Intestinal polyposisi with melanin pigmentation.

Etiology

Is Unknown. It is inherited a an autosomal dominant trait.

Clinical Features

Skin

There are numerous, usually descrete, brown to bluish balc macules on skin, especially about the facial orifices-perioral, perinasal and periorbital. The macules range from 1 to 5 mm in diameter. The pigmentation is usually present from birth and seems to fade somewhat at bout puberty.

Gastrointestinal System

Polyposis of gastrointestinal tract is clinically more important component of the syndrome. The polyps are probably hamartomatous in origin, and have a very low malignant potential.

Bartholomew and Dahlin suggested the following sites to be involved in percentage as jejunum 63% ileum 55%; large bowel and rectum 36% each; stomach 23%, duodenum 15% and appendix 3%.

Thus the polyps may befound any whee in the mucous secreting protion of gastrointestinal tract. So these patients have frequent episodes of abdominal pain and signs of minor obstruction.

The polyps are usually described as bening adenomatous tumors varying in size from 0.5 to 0.7 cm in diameter.

Oral Manifestations

On the lips, especially the lower lip and on oral mucosa rounde, oval or irregular, rarely, confluent macules of bluish-gray pigment of variable intensity may be seen. These are somewhat larger than those on skin, about 1 to 12 mm in size. They also involved buccal mucosa and less frequently palate, gingiva and floor of the mouth.

The facial pigment tends to fade later in life, but the mucosal pigmentation persists.

PIERRE ROBIN SYNDROME

Synonyms

Robin Anomalad.

Etiology

Exact etioloty is unknown etiology is unknown. Its thought to be due to malposition and interposition of the tongue between the palatal shelves. Arrest of kandibular development may prevent descent of the tongue and failure ofpalatal helf elevation and fusion. Recent evidences suggest that the primary defect may be due to genetically influenced metabolic growth disturbances of the maxilla and mandible rather than to mechanical obstruction by the tongue, during embryogenesis.

Clinical Features

Oral Manifestations

Oral changes are the most evident ones in this syndrome. It consists of micrognathia, cleft alate, and glossoptosis. In this syndrome, the primary defect is hypoplasia of mandible which prevents the normal descent of the developing tongue between the medially growing palatalshelves resulting in cleft-plate. Because of this mechanism cleft lip does not occur in association with cleftpalate. The hypoplastic mandible, characteristically produces "bird facies". The most important result of this jaw malformation is respiratory and feeding difficulties, although exact explanation of its occurrence is uncertain, The usual suggestion is that failure of support of tongue musculature occurs because of the micrognathia, allowing the tongue to fall down and backward, partially obstructing epiglottis. Feeding problems are though to be due to inadequate control of the rongue.

Usually these patients have difficulty during the inspiratory phase of respiration with periodic cyanotic attacks. The tongue acts as a ball valve preventing inhalation but allowing exhalation.

Face

Iti s typically described as "Birds facies" or "Andy Gump" appearance. About 20% of the patients are mentally retarded. There can also be congenital heart defects like patent ductus arteriosus and foramen ovale; auricular septal defect and coarctation of aorta.

Treatment

No specific treatment.

PLUMMER-VINSON SYNDROME

Synonyms

Paterson-Kelly syndrome; Hysterical dysphagia; Sideropenic dysphagia.

Etiology

Iron deficiency is the primary cause of the syndrome. Chronic blood loss (as in profuse menstruation), inadequate dietry intake, faulty iron absorption or increased requirements of iron can lead to iron deficiency.

Clinical Features

Plumm-erVinson Syndrome occurs chiefly in women in fourth to fift decades of life.

Oral manifestations

Cracks or fissures at the corner of the mouth; the vermilion border of the lip is thinned and mouth is narrowed. The tongue is smooth, devoid of papillae, and usually red in color, it is often painful and edematous. Leukoplakia of the oral mucosa has been reported in a number of cases, especially on the dorsum of tongue.

Other Manifestations

General Appearance

The facila skin is usually pale, dry, smooth and atrophic, giving the patient a characteristic ashtenic appearance. The nails are brittle and spoon shaped (koilonychias)

Esophaus

Dysphagia is the outstanding feature. The difficulty in swallowing is attributed to formation esophageal stricture or web; which occurs at third or sixth cervical vertebrae. The web is described as a thin, crescentic membrane arising usually from the anterior esophageal wall.

The mucous membrane of oral cavity and esophagus are atrophic and show loss of normal keratinization. The atrophy of mucous membranes of upper alimentary tract predisposes to the development of carcinoma (therefore it is a precancerous condition.)

Laboratory Findings

Blood examination reveals a hypochromic microcytic anaemi, bh% is low, and there is absence of free hydrochloric acid in the stomach. So conversion of ferric iron to ferrous iron is prevented. The esophageal web can be demonstrated radiologically by barium swallow or esophagoscopy.

Treatment

The syndrome responds to iron therapy and high protein diet.

REITER'S SYNDROME

Synonyms

Conjunctival-urethral-synovial syndrome; Non gonococal urethritis with conjunctivitis and arthritis.

Etiology

The etiology is still unclear. There is evidence of infectious origin. In recent years pelurophenumonia like organisms (PPLO) have been implicated and even more recently, a Bedsonia group of virus has been isolated from the patents. An abnormal immune response to microbial antigens is regarded as a likely mechanism for multiple manifestations of this syndrome.

Clinical Features

Iti s most commonly occurring in men between the age group of 20 to 30 years. Above the age of 50, the disease is seldom seen. There is typical tetrad of manifestations -
- Urethritis
- Arthritis
- Conjunctivitis and
- Mucocutaneous lesions

The onset of symptoms may be preceded by weight loss, fatigability and diarrhea. The urethritis generally precedes the appearance of other lesions. The urethral involvement consists of discharge associated with itching and burning sensation. The examination if discharge reveals no bacteria.

Arthritis

In almost all of the cases there is polyarticular involvement, and the weight bearing joints are commonly affected.

Conjunctivitis

It is usually bilateral and is often so mild that the condition is overlooked. The initial symptoms of conjunctivitis include photophobia, epiphora and then redness of conjunctiva and mucopurarulent discharge.

Skin

The lesions are similar to kerotosis blennorrhagica, and are found on palms and soles and occasionally on trunk. The skin manifestation consists of red or yellow keratotic macules pr papules which eventually desquamate.

Oral Manifestations

The oral lesions are described as aphthous type ulcerations by Pindborg which are usually painless, red, slightly elevated areas, sometimes granular or even vesicular, with a white circinate border. The lesions can occur any where in oral cavity. The gongue may exhibit superficial erosions similar to that of geographic tongue.

Treatment

The disease may undergo spontaneous remission. Non-steroidal, anti inflammatory drugs, antibiotics and steroids can be used.

SJOGREN'S SYNDROME

Synonyms

Sicca syndrome; Gougerot-Mickulics-Sjogren syndrome; Secreto-inhibitor syndrome.

It was first described in detail by Henrek Sjogren ion 1933.

Sjogren's syndrome is a condition originally described as a triad consisting of keratoconjunctivitis sica, xerostomia and rheumatoid arthritis.

Primary Sogrens syndrome (SS) affects the exocrine glands only, primarily the lacrimal and salivary glands. Secondary SS consists of lacrimal and salivary gland involvement with an associated connective tissue disease (like systemic lupus erythematosus, polyarteritis nodosa, scleroderma and rheumatoid arthritis).

Etiology

Various causes have been suggested-genetic, hormonal, infectious and immunologic. Now most authorities sugest autoimmune to be the cause, as 75% of the patients had in their sera anti salivary duct antibody (study by Bertram). A similar antibody was found in the sera of 24% of paeitnes with systemic lupus erythematosus.

The trigger for abnormal immune response is unknown, but some investigators believe that viruses particularly EB or type A retrovisus, may play an initiating role.

Clnical Features

It occurs commonly in females after 40 years of age, although children or young adults may be affected. The female male ratio is round 10:1.

Oral Manifestations

Xerostomia or dryness of mouth was the chief complaint of about 82% of patients, (in a study by Daniels and colleagues) but the history of salivary gland varies. The dry mouth may be accompanied by bilateral enlargement of parotid glands, unilateral enlargement or no enlargement. Enlargement of submandibular glands may also occur. Absence of salivary gland enlargement does not exclude SS as a possible cause of xerostomia. Because of dryness of mouth, patient complains of inability to chew, swallow or wear dentures. There is severe burning sensation of oral mucosa. The lack of oral secretion may lead to secondary oral diseases such as candidiasis or an increase in dental caries. The color of mucosa may vary from pale pink to fiery red. The tongue may be depapillated and so appears smooth and lobulated.

Eyes

Dryness and burning sensation are the main complaints. The corneal epithelium is thinner than normal patients complain of continued feeling of dirt or other foreign body in the eye. The symptoms are caused by failure of lacrimal and conjunctival glands to maintain adequate secretion. Continuous severe, lacrimal gland involvement may lead to corneal ulceration and conjunctivitis.

Other Mucous Membranes

Dryness of larynx, pharynx and nose is noted by some patients. Lack of secretions in upper respiratory tract, may lead to pneumonia. There can also be dryness of vagina.

Other symptoms

Other signs of secondary SS depends chiefly on associated collagen disease and include a wide variety of joint, muscle and skin findings seen in rheumatoid arthritis, Scleroderma, SLE. Characteristic generalized manifestation of primary SS include renal involvement, polyneuropathy, vasculitis and pneumonitis.

Laboratory Aids

Histologically

Ther are three types of histologic alterations in major salivary glands described.

- One   - There may be intense lymphocytic infiltration of the gland replacing all acinar structures, although the lobular architecture is preserved. The lymphocytes have been shown to be predominantely T helper memory cells, which are believed to trigger the B lymphocyte hyperactivity associated with SS.
- Two   - Ther may be proliferation of ductal epithelium and myoepithelium to form "epithelimyopithelial islands".
- Three   - Atrophy of the glands sequential to lymphocytic infilteration.

Salivary Gland Functions

Can be measured by three tests – Salivary flow rate, minor salivary gland biopsy and salivary scintigraphy.

Salivary Flow Rate

Can be accomplished by placing a Lashly, Carlson Critenden or other specifically fabricated cup over Stenen's duct orifice. The salivary glands can be stinulated by lemon juice every 30 secs for

10 mins. The normal rane being 5 ml secretion per gland, if flow is below 0.5 ml, it can be considered as SS.

Minor Salivary Gland Biopsy

This is most specific and widely used. It this technique, a 2.0 cm incision is made on lower labial mucosa. A minimum of 5 gland lobules are removed and lymphocyte focus scroes are determined by counting the number of chronic inflammatory foci cells per 4 mm^3 of specimen. Changes are graded from 0 to 4. Investigations using immuno histologic techniques demonstrate that the presence of immunoglobin A and G containing cells is a more accurate measure of SS than lymphocyte focus scores.

Sequential Salivary Scientigraphy

It consists of recording the uptake, concentration and excretion of Tc-pertechnate by the salivary glands using a Y-scintillation camera. Ten millicuries of radioactive isotope is injected intravenously. Photographs are taken every 2 mins for first 10 mins and then every 10 mins for 1 hour. SS patients demonstrate a decrease in total uptake of the isotope by the salivary glands; slow uptake, or slow excretion of the isotope into saliva.

Sailography may be of diagnostic value but is no longer considred desirabl,e as there is some danger of glandular damage by the injected dye, and also in patients with severe SS, the dye will remain in the glands interfering with further tests. Sailographs demonstrate the formation of punctuate, cavity defects which are filled with radiopaque contrast media. This produces "Cherry blossom" or "branch less fruit-laden tree" effect radiographically.

MRI is not invasive and may be a useful method of distinguishing salivary glands enlarged due to SS, from other salivary gland disorders. A "salt and pepper" appearance of the glands on MRI is particularly suggestive of Sjogren's Syndrome.

Optholmologists use three tests – to evaluate lacrimal gland function;

- Schirmer's test – It consists of palcing a filter paper strip in lower conjunctival sac. Normal patients will wet 15 mm of filter paper in 5 mins. Patients with SS will we less tan 5 mm of paper.
- Brakup time test (BUT)- Is performed using a slit lamp and noting the interval between a complete blink and the appearance of dry spot on the cornea.
- Rose Bengal dye test- Is used to detect damaged and denuded areas of the cornea.

Treatment

There is no satisfactory treatment for SS. The goal of treatemtn is to minimize the secondary effects of decreased exocrine secretion. Keratoconjunctivitis is treated by instillation of ocular lubricants such as artificial tears containing methyl cellulose, and xerostomia is treated by saliva substitute and use of pilocarpine-a muscaranic cholinergic agonist agent, 5 mg 3 to 4 times daily. Patients at risk of developing pneumococcol pneumonia due to decreased tracheobronchial secretions should be vaccinated against common strains of pneumococci.

Dental caries-should be controlled and daily home use of topical fluorides and frequent oral hygiene visits, which include fluoride treatment will decrease caries rate. Oral candidiasis can be managed by topical application of nystatin.

STEVENS-JOHNSON SYNDROME

Synonyms

Fiessinger-Rendu syndrome.

Etiology

Is unknown. The most common precipitating agent discussed by shelley is herpes simplex infection, preceding the disease by one to three weeks. Certain bacterial and fungal infections and certain druds like barbiturates, phenyl butazone, penicillins etc. may also trigger the disease.

Clinical Features

It is a severe, bullous form of erythema multiform, with wide spread involvement of skin, oral cavity, eyes and genitalia.

It affects males more frequently than females and occurs in young adults.

Skin manifestations

It is characterized by occurrence of asymptomatic, vividly erythematous discrete maculaes, papules or vesicles and bullae distributed in symmetrical pattern over the hands, arms, feet, leg, face and neck. The individual lesions may vary in size and are generally a few centimeter less in diameter.

A concentric ring like appearance of the lesions, resulting from the varying shades of erythema, giving rise to 'target', 'iris', or 'bull's eye' appearance, consisting of a central bulla or pale clearing area surrounded by edema and bands of erythema.

Oral Manifestations

Oral Manifestations

Oral lesions commonly appear along with skin lesing in the approximately 45% of cases. In some cases oral lesions are predominant or single sign of disease.

The oral lesions may be found on lips, buccal mucosa, gingival, tongue and palate. The initial stage in the development of oral lesion is a small erythematous plaque soon followed by a vesicle or bulla, which ruptures forming shallow erosions covered by necrotic exudates or pseudomembrane. The lips may exhibit ulceration with bloody cursting and are painful.

Ocular Manifestations

Conjunctivitis, corneal ulceration and panophthalmitis are seen. Blindness may result chiefly from recurrent bacterial infection.

Genital Lesions

Consists of non specific urethristis, balanitis and or vaginal ulcers.

It can also affect respiratory tract leading to tracheobronchial ulceration and pneumonia.

Histological Features

The histologic picture is not of diagnostic value. The cutaneous or mucosal lesions generally exhibit intracellular edema of spinous layer of epithelium and edema of the superficial connective tissue which may produce subepidermal vesicle. In study of oral lesions, *Shklar* has described a zone of severe liquefaction degeneration in upper layers of epithelium, intraepithelial vesicle formation of inflammatory cell infiltrate, chiefly lymphocytes and often neutrophils and eosinophils are also present.

Treatemnt

Usually treatment with supportive measures including topical anaesthetic mouth washes and a soft or liquid diet. If symptoms does not respond, then a short course of corticosteroids is administered 30 mg to 50 mg/day.

STURGE-WEBER SYNDROME

Synonyms

Encephalotrigeminal angiomatosis; ncephalo facial angiomatosis; Sturge-Kalischer Weber syndrome.

It is characterized by – venous agngioma of the leptomeninges overlying the cerebral cortex with ipsilateral angiomatous lesions of the face, ipsilateral syriform calcifications of brain, epilepsy, mental retardation, contralateral hemiplegia and ocular involvement.

Etiology

Etiology is unknown. Genetic predisposition seems to play no role.

Clinical Features

Brain

Angioma of the leptomeninges seen over the posterior parietal and occipital lobes. The angiomatosis consists of thin walled venous vessels. Characteristic feature of the syndrome is the intracranial, convolutional ,gyriform calcification, which presents as double contoured lines. The "tram-line" calcification is pathognomic on radiograph.

Face

Ipsilateral cerebral angiomatosis a nevus flammeus (port wine nevus) commonly occurs on the face. Facial nevus is present at birth and in most cases, it is unilateral. The color varies from pink to purplish red. A decrease in intensity of color with inceasing age has been noted. Cushing noted a correlation between the distribution of port wine nevus and the course of trigemal nerve.

Nervous System

Epilepsy is common and symptoms appear in infancy. The seizures are contralateral to the angiomatosis, and most often are focal, but generalized convulsions may also occur. Hemiparesis occurs less frequently.

Eyes

The classic ophthalmologic lesion is a choroidal angioma. Bupthalmos and glaucoma are also frequently found.

Oral Manifestations

The most frequent oral symptoms is involvement of oral mucosa. Angiomatous lesions may involve cheeks and lips less frequently palate is also involvew. The tongue may be affected, showing either telangiectasia or hemihypertrophy. The ipsilateral alveolar precess in the maxilla may be hypertrophic, with diastema of the teeth. About 1/3rd of the patients are mentally retarded.

Treatement

The treatment is a neurosurgical problem, although convulsions can sometimes be controlled by anticonvulsant drugs.

TREACHER COLLINS SYNDROME
Synonyms

Mandibulofacial dysostosis; Franceschetti Zwahlen-klein Syndrome; Bilateral facial agenesis. Although the syndrome was first described by Thomson in 1846-47, the credit is usually given to Berry or to Treacher Collins, Who described the essential components of the syndrome.

The syndrome is inherited as an autosomal dominant trait. Authors classified syndrome into several forms complete, incomplete, abortive, unilateral and atypical.

Etiology

Tfhe theories of origin of this syndrome have been numerous and have been revived by Synyder. The concept of Mann and Kilner based on embryological considerations, suggests that the developmental disturbances occurs at about 50 mm stage or towards the end of second month of fetal life. Hovels indicated that causative factor was maldevelopmkent of head neural crest.

Clinical Features

Oral Manifestations

Include hypoplasia of facial bones especially of the malar bones and mandible. Macrostomia, high palate (some times cleft) abnormal position and malocclusion of the teeth.

Other Features

Facies

The facial appearance is characteristic with downwards slopin palpebral fissures, depressed cheek bones, deformed pinna, receding chin and large fish like mouth. A typcal hair growth in the in the form of gongue shaped process of the hair line extending towards the cheeks is seen.

Eyes

Though vision is usually normal, the palpebral fissures slope laterally downward (antimongoloid obliquity) and often there is a coloboma in the outer third of the lower lid. Deficiency of eye lashes, and sometimes the upper lids is encountered.

Ears

Pinna is often deformed, crumpled forward, or misplaced. There is also malformation of middle and internal ears.

Nose

The nasal-frontal angle is usually obliterated and the bridge of nose is raised. The nose appears large because of lack of malar development. There are blind fistulas between the angles of the ears and the angles of the mouth. Most of the patients are mentally retarded.

Treatement

Ther is is no treatment for this conditions, but the prognosis is good.

TROTTER'S SYNDROME

Synonyms

Sinus of Morgagni Syndrome.

It was first described by Trotter in 1911. The syndrome is seen most often in male during third to fourth decades of life.

Etiology

The syndrome results from invasion of the latgeral wall of nasopharynx (sinus of Morgagni) by a tumor, usually anaplastic carcinoma.

Clinical Features

Unilateral deafness (as the tumor extends, it compresses the Eustachian tube). Pain over the area supplied by mandibular division (Temporal area, ear, lower jaw, teeth, tongue and anesthesia over the mental area) Trigeminal nerve.

Ipsilateral defective mobility of the palate (as the tumor invades the palatal musculature). Trismus (results as the tumor extends into pterygoids).

TURNER'S SYNDROME

Synonyms

Xo syndrome; Gonadal dysgenesis or agenesis, Overian short stature syndrome; Genital dwarfism. The syndrome was described by Turner in 1938. The cause is not known. Only 45 chromosomes ar present. Loss of one of the x-chrmososmes produces xo syndrome.

Clinical Features

Oral Manifestations
Two of the most constant oral findings are high palatal vault and hypoplastic mandible. Cleft palate has also been noted. The mouth has also been found to be small, with the corners pulled down by pterygium colli, producing characteristic sphinx like visage.

Other Manifestations

Include short stature (50-58 inches), primary amenorrhea, infantile uterus, infantile vagina and breasts, ovasrian agenesis, pterygium colli and low hair line at back of the neck.

Mental retardation, deafness, coarctation of aorta, deformation of nails and ears are other features.

www.ingramcontent.com/pod-product-compliance
Lightning Source LLC
Chambersburg PA
CBHW051800170526
45167CB00005B/1814